Representations of HIV and AIDS

MANCHESTER
UNIVERSITY PRESS

To Simon, of course

Representations
of HIV and AIDS
Visibility blue/s

GABRIELE GRIFFIN

Manchester University Press
Manchester and New York

distributed exclusively in the USA by St. Martin's Press

Published by Manchester University Press
Oxford Road, Manchester M13 9NR, UK
and Room 400, 175 Fifth Avenue, New York, NY 10010, USA
http://www.manchesteruniversitypress.co.uk

Distributed exclusively in the USA by
St. Martin's Press, Inc., 175 Fifth Avenue, New York,
NY 10010, USA

Distributed exclusively in Canada by
UBC Press, University of British Columbia, 2029 West Mall,
Vancouver, BC, Canada V6T 1Z2

British Library Cataloguing-in-Publication Data
A catalogue record for this book is available from the British Library

Library of Congress Cataloging-in-Publication Data applied for

ISBN 0 7190 4710 2 *hardback*
     0 7190 4711 0 *paperback*

First published 2000

07 06 05 04 03 02 01 00   10 9 8 7 6 5 4 3 2 1

Typeset in Walbaum with Futura display by Northern Phototypesetting Co. Ltd, Bolton
Printed in Great Britain
by Bookcraft (Bath) Ltd, Midsomer Norton

Contents

Illustrations

Acknowledgements

Kingston University gave me a sabbatical upon arrival to complete this book, for which I am very grateful. I would also like to thank Simon Raw, Press and PR Officer of the Haymarket Theatre, Leicester, for supplying me with copies of reviews of the Haymarket's production of *The Destiny of Me*. Further thanks go to Della Hirons of the Terrence Higgins Trust whose archive proved to be an invaluable resource. Matthew Frost of Manchester University Press was supportive throughout and prompt and helpful in all his advice and dealings with me. My thanks go to him, too.

The poet and writer Suniti Namjoshi kindly granted permission to reproduce her poem 'I give her the rose'. The photographer Richard Sawdon Smith generously gave permission to publish his photograph *Portrait of Simon*, also known as *Simon 68–97*, for which he won the Kobal Portrait Prize in 1997. Douglas Crimp wrote a nice email, and gave permission to reproduce images from *AIDSdemographics* (Seattle, Bay Press, 1990). The Health Education Authority granted permission to reproduce images from their campaigns promoting safer sex. Bloodaxe Books gave permission to reproduce lines from Jackie Kay's volumes of poetry *The Adoption Papers* (1991) and *Off Colour* (1998).

A previous version of Chapter 5, 'Alien bodies – HIV/AIDS in Jackie Kay's poetry', appeared in *Kicking Daffodils: Twentieth-century Women Poets* (ed. V. Bertram, Edinburgh, Edinburgh University Press, 1997); and previous versions of Chapter 7, 'Safe and sexy? Lesbian erotica in the age of AIDS' were published in *Romance Revisited* (eds L. Pearce and J. Stacey, London, Lawrence and Wishart, 1995) and in the *Canadian Woman Studies* journal (spring 1996).

Many people were involved in the making of this book, offering support and advice both directly and indirectly, and in many different ways. I would like to thank them all. They include Anjona Roy, Chris Bainton, Gill Perkins, Josie Pedersen, Clair Roberts, Tricia Connell, Al Garthwaite, Lisa Price, Jalna Hanmer, Stevi Jackson, Sasha Roseneil, Hanna Zielke, Katrin Zielke, Christiane Beer, John Lynch, Andrea Zielke, Julia Bush, Lynn Aitken, George Savona, Elaine Aston, Greg Woods, Andrew Stephenson and many others. To all of you, my thanks.

Introduction

> the structure and stability of contemporary configurations of heterosexuality require the invisibility and interdiction of same-sex desire while the fight against AIDS historically required that the lives of those framed by such desire be made both visible and legitimate. (Yingling 1991: 300)

I began thinking about this book in the early 1990s. As I realize now, HIV/AIDS was at the height of its public visibility at that time, signalled by the proliferation of its cultural (re)presentation. New films, plays, videos and other visually over-determined cultural productions centring on HIV/AIDS were still regularly appearing then but, as I discuss briefly in Chapter 1, in the town where I lived then, for example, audience numbers were dwindling. When I went to see Derek Jarman's film *Blue* in 1993, only a handful of people attended the film during its short run in the local alternative arts venue. Larry Kramer's *The Destiny of Me*, performed at the local theatre in the same year (1993), had to close early owing to low audience figures, even though it featured stars such as Simon Callow and Patty Boulaye. However, even despite these dwindling audience numbers in at least some locations, in the early 1990s HIV/AIDS was at the height of its public visibility. This is registered in this volume through the fact that both Chapter 1 and the Conclusion centre on films which first appeared in 1993: Derek Jarman's *Blue* and Jonathan Demme's *Philadelphia*. The public visibility I refer to here relates to the fact that between about 1988 and 1993 a steady accumulation of visually based work and interventions had been produced both by AIDS activists and, increasingly for a time, by mainstream institutions. This work included art (both 'high' and 'low'),[1] installations, photography exhibitions, videos and films, health promotion campaigns based on posters and mass media publications, as well as images of people with HIV/AIDS produced as part of its media coverage. A form of cultural accretion, it had generated a public awareness of HIV/AIDS (and often misinformation) by its cumulative presence which, as I argue in the Conclusion, is no longer prominent. However, in the early 1990s there was a strong sense that HIV/AIDS was here to stay, that the numbers of those infected with HIV and suffering from AIDS-related diseases were on the increase, and that the impact of HIV/AIDS in the cultural arena was sustained and significant in raising and changing public awareness, if not always public understanding in its two senses of knowledge and empathy, of HIV/AIDS.

Lesbians and HIV/AIDS

My thinking about *Representations of HIV and AIDS: Visibility blue/s* was informed by a variety of debates and issues which occurred or arose in the early 1990s, and which became significant for and are reflected in the book's title and content. The first of these was discussions amongst lesbians about the appropriateness of lesbians becoming involved in struggles around HIV/AIDS, still perceived by many as effectively a gay men's disease, instead of expanding our energies on issues and concerns directly and primarily affecting lesbians and women. From a radical or a separatist lesbian feminist perspective, becoming involved in what was perceived to be a men's issue (even if these men were gay) was viewed as a misguided act, replicating notions of femininity associated with caring, nurturing[2] and subservience to men's lives and preoccupations which lesbians and women[3] had spent a long time struggling against. Questions were raised such as, 'Can you imagine gay men rallying around lesbian issues such as breast cancer?' and 'What have we in common with men whose lifestyles [speak: their sexual behaviours and patterns] are all about quick gratification?'[4]. There was also a strong sense that lesbians had far fewer resources than gay men,[5] often working in the service and caring industries rather than at the designer end of the market, and that we could not afford to have these few resources dissipated through investment in men. And, finally, or perhaps foremostly, it was felt that lesbians were unlikely to become infected with HIV and develop AIDS.[6]

These concerns are understandable even though they ignored the fact that HIV/AIDS is not only, and was not even then only, a gay men's issue, and the fact that lesbians had been involved from the beginning in the struggle against HIV/AIDS since it affected people we knew directly and since it was enmeshed with struggles around visibility politics which had been, and had become, increasingly important as part of the struggle for the advancement of lesbian and gay rights. Many lesbians, however, felt themselves to be invisibilized by the foregrounding of HIV/AIDS as the main agenda item in the fight for lesbian and gay rights. They took the view that as men in mainstream, heteronormative culture determined political and other agendas, so, in the lesbian and gay communities, men's concerns dictated where energies and resources were invested.[7] Associated with these discussions were the debates about lesbian sexuality itself, and the rise in the cultural production from the 1980s onwards of lesbian erotica/porn which in turn raised questions about whether or not and how HIV/AIDS was to be dealt with in contexts like representations of lesbian sado-masochism which advocated sexual practices that might promote HIV infection. These issues are dealt with in Chapter 7.

Blue, mourning and militancy

The second experience which was crucial to the writing of this book was going to see Derek Jarman's *Blue*. This film is the focus of Chapter 1, and the title of this book owes much to *Blue*. In that film Jarman, the man whose penchant for detail and enjoyment of intricacy was evident in all his work, his writing, his art, his films, indeed his famous garden at Dungeness,[8] created a work in which that detail, usually stunningly presented at the visual level, was unexpectedly and strikingly transposed into a preoccupation with the details of the auditory world in the face of Jarman's failing sight, a function of his suffering from AIDS. Since film is in the first instance a visual medium, the specificity of what can be seen in Jarman's film, the continuous blue offered to the viewer, acts as a confounding reverse discourse to both the usual cinematic experience of watching a film and to the mainstream images of those suffering from AIDS that dominated the mass media. The word *blue/s* in this book's title is thus in part a reference to that experience and to that film.

Blue is in some respects elegaic,[9] a lament for many things lost, for some of Jarman's friends who succumbed to AIDS-related illnesses before him, for his own physical decline, for the sufferings of the gay community over time. But this mourning is also interrupted by poetic passages which are celebratory and affirmative, which refuse any stance of self-pity or victimization. Jarman's work, and this goes for *Blue*, too, is a site of resistance to the homophobia which he had experienced himself and which inflected, and continues to inflect, much of the public response to HIV/AIDS. In that respect, Jarman made a representation in and with *Blue*, which sought to intervene in the orthodoxies and entrenched opinions that were beginning to make themselves felt in perceptions around HIV/AIDS in public contexts. That representation was a protest as much as a testimony, and it is partly in answer to this that I use the term 'representation' in the title of this book.

Representation is both about cultural (re)production and imaging, *and* about the desire to create a presence, to achieve visibility and recognition, to participate, including in public debates and fora. It is about representing or being represented, in the political as much as in the cultural sense. In fact, as I discuss in Chapter 2, which centres on *AIDS-demographics* and the work of ACT UP, it is through representation and being represented at the cultural level that gay men in particular have sought to achieve political representation in the face of the HIV/AIDS epidemic. The two, cultural and political representation, are thus intertwined and that in ways which are complex, sometimes contradictory, and fraught with difficulties for those seeking to utilize them effectively to generate social and political change. As Piontek put it in 1992: 'there is no cultural consensus concerning the meaning of AIDS, and the significance of the epidemic remains contested even today, two years into the second decade of the epidemic' (144).

That lack of consensus was due to several factors. It was partly a function of the 'nature' of the epidemic which saw changes in perception both around who was affected by it and around how best to deal with it, issues which are addressed in several of the chapters in this volume but in particular in chapters 2 and 3. It was also a function of debates amongst diverse groups of people about how best to raise awareness concerning HIV/AIDS. AIDS activists emerging from the gay communities in the USA and in the UK engaged in discussions about the efficacy of different forms of cultural interventions. Some were predominantly concerned with generating resources for research into HIV/AIDS and for support of those infected with HIV and/or dying from AIDS-related diseases. Others found the sudden flood of deaths of close friends so overwhelming that they wanted to be able, in the first instance, to mourn their losses publicly and have their grief acknowledged. 'Mourning and militancy', the title of a key article on this issue by Douglas Crimp (1989b), became the bywords of these debates which were part of the lack of cultural consensus referred to by Piontek. Eventually, they also became part of the discussions around what one might term 'the ownership' of HIV/AIDS discourses, that is part of the question of who was entitled to, and/or should, speak for, indeed represent those affected by HIV/AIDS and how. I use ownership' here not as a pejorative term but to signal the deeply held views by many of the communities they represent, whether these be gay, or poor, or from diverse ethnic communities, that the HIV/AIDS agenda was hijacked or taken over by particular groups of people with their own interests at heart and with the result that others in consequence lost out, particularly if the groups in question, who had achieved representation, managed to marshal resources which others felt were (more) urgently needed amongst their own communities. In some respects, Oppenheimer and Reckitt's (1997) *Acting on AIDS* is a testimony to that phenomenon, pointing to the difficulties of being just and equitable in a situation of great injustice, affecting many and very different people,[10] some of whom have better, and are more capable of accessing, both cultural and political representation than others. In Chapters 2 and 3 in particular I discuss some of the issues and conflicts that arose as both cultural and political representation were sought by different people affected by, and dealing with, HIV/AIDS.

Visuality and visibility

A third, related question which fuelled the writing of this book was why a visually under-determined condition, if I might use the term 'condition' here, such as HIV/AIDS, surfaced culturally in the first instance particularly prominently in visually over-determined media like films, posters, theatre pieces, installations, art exhibitions and videos. No parallel cultural proliferation can be found for other conditions which are in some respects similar, such as cancer, for example.[11] There are several answers to this questions which emerge in the course of this volume. One answer, not sufficient or exhaustive, lies in the ways in which HIV/AIDS emerged or became visible, its sudden appearance and speed of spread which necessitated speed of response in media that could reach large audiences quickly such as television and billboards. Vast numbers of people were dying unexpectedly and quickly; this seemingly unprecedented experience[12] necessitated swift responses to elicit intervention and change. Another answer, also neither sufficient nor exhaustive, relates to the indeterminancy of HIV/AIDS, meaning the inability of medical and socio-political bodies to fix HIV/AIDS unambiguously to particular groups, behaviours or patterns of manifestation. In the absence of such specificities there were perceived needs both by the mainstream media and by AIDS activists to project images related to HIV/AIDS which 'captured' the realities of the situation as it emerged and changed. As suggested in Chapters 2 and 3, the different agendas which drove mainstream media and AIDS activists resulted in very different kinds of representations and images. AIDS activists fought hard to counteract the distorting representations of HIV/AIDS fed to the 'general public' by the mainstream media.[13] The visual field became a ground on which battles about HIV/AIDS representation were fought, not only between diverse communities but also, as Chapter 3 indicates, within communities such as the gay community. But utilizing the visual field to project messages about HIV/AIDS was also a means of visibilizing HIV/AIDS, of generating public space for it when governments were slow to respond to the threats posed by HIV/AIDS. Finally, and still neither sufficiently nor exhaustively, it was a means of externalizing, visibilizing and objectifying[14] the grief experienced by those losing friends and relatives to HIV/AIDS.

The primacy of the word

One of the striking aspects of the visual representations centring on HIV/AIDS was their logocentricity. Only in the context of high art (see Chapter 3) was the visual field sometimes given over to images which had no words other than a title such as 'Untitled'. In the fight against HIV/AIDS, the visual arena thus became the means to message but the message itself was virtually never purely visual. Indeed, where it was, as in certain high art forms, it generated an indeterminacy or ambiguity of meaning which effectively dissociated the image from HIV/AIDS thus potentially voiding it of its HIV/AIDS-related impact. As I discuss in Chapter 2, much activist art, in contrast to certain certain types of 'high art', used text *as* image in order to specify its meaning, or a combination of text and image. Such visualization was driven by the need to generate an instant and unambiguous impact. Clear, brief and therefore memorable slogans were designed to influence public opinion and change public behaviour. This was as true of the activist art of ACT UP as it was of some of the health promotion campaigns discussed in Chapter 3. Both activist art and health promotion campaigns aimed at intervention and change at a time when mourning those who had been lost through HIV/AIDS was also (still) very much in the public eye.

Unmarked: bodies that matter

As the means of mourning those lost to HIV/AIDS, representations in the visual field and public spectacle became the perhaps most sustainedly theorized interventions in the visual field taken up by cultural theorists in their analysis of HIV/AIDS. A further and important influence on the writing of this volume was thus certain theoretical writings on HIV/AIDS which were published in the early 1990s, and in particular the work of two feminist cultural theorists, Judith Butler and Peggy Phelan. The year 1993 seemed like a time when bodies did not appear to matter very much at all, 'bodies' here understood both as the physical body as a previously essentialized corporeality and bodies as regards the sheer numbers of people dying from AIDS which did not seem to galvanize governments significantly into decisive action to intervene in the mounting HIV/AIDS crisis. Just when one might well have wanted to ask, what matter bodies?, Butler published *Bodies that Matter.*[15] Towards the end of this volume she began to address the issue of public mourning and its relation to gender, sexuality and heteronormativity, attempting to account for the ways in which homosexuals had begun to intervene culturally in the indifference of governments towards those affected by HIV/AIDS through enacting their rage, anger and grief in a range of cultural forms. These cultural forms were both highly visual and performative. Butler's text articulated what seems to me to have been the dominant sense of the early 1990s in relation to HIV/AIDS: mourning of those lost, and frustration at the lack of government intervention in seeking to halt the epidemic.

Similarly, Phelan's *Unmarked* (1993) considered the impact of HIV/AIDS on visual and performative cultures but the driver of her text was the problematization of the visibility politics which was informing gay and lesbian activism. Phelan suggested that in contrast to the notion that visibility, and the disruption of mainstream consensus through the positing of counter-images, was an effective means for political representation and gaining access to power, it encouraged surveillance and divisions which might not benefit those seeking to intervene politically in order to improve their situation. Phelan argued that the reason for this lay in the relationship between representation and the real. Quoting Butler she suggested that 'the real is positioned both before and after its representation; and representation becomes a moment of the reproduction and consolidation of the real' (Phelan 1993: 2). Since 'the real is read through representation, and representation is read through the real, each representation relies on and reproduces a specific logic of the real; this logical real promotes its own representation' (Phelan 1993: 2). Phelan cites various examples of different kinds of 'real' such as the legal real or various types of psychoanalytic real and asserts that 'each of these concepts of the real contains within it a meta-text of exclusionary power. Each real believes itself to be the Real-real' (1993: 3). In other words, these diverse concepts of the real, generated within different discourses, constitute contestations of the meaning of the real at the same time that they lay claim to their specific meaning as the 'truth'. Phelan argues that 'the visible itself is woven into each of these discourses [of the real] as an unmarked conspirator in the maintenance of each discursive real' (3) and that, and this is crucial here, 'the visible real is employed as a truth effect for the establishment of these discursive and representational notions of the real' (3). Since the visible real is a truth effect, that is it is never 'the real thing' but always an effect of a particular truth claim, cultural representation both conceals and reveals a real which reinforces notions of difference as 'real' differences, thus maintaining the gap between 'them' and 'us' which has always served as a means of abjecting those perceived to be other. The visible real is a truth effect because it arises, as Butler puts it, through the 'forcible citation of a norm' (1993: 232). Diverse forms of visual culture, whether these be theatre or film or other kinds of images and imagings, are objects of conventions which make these a 'bounded "act"' (Butler 1993: 234) in which the norms or conventions of the specific cultural form 'precede, constrain, and exceed the performer' (Butler 1993: 234). To the extent that these norms and conventions rely on and reproduce the logic of the real as constituted by dominant society for example, they defy intentions to intervene in that society, to challenge and change the representations dominant within that society. This is evident in my discussion of Randy Shilts's *And the Band Played On* in Chapter 4 and in my analysis of Larry Kramer's theatre works *The Normal Heart* and *The Destiny of Me* in Chapter 6. Where Jarman's *Blue* refuses mainstream cinematic conventions and the conventional imaging of bodies suffering from AIDS-related illnesses, Shilts and Kramer utilize certain mainstream representational conventions, thus generating very different effects from the ones achieved by Jarman. Phelan (1993) calls for changes in representational strategies to counter the truth effects or forcible citations of norms or conventions referred to above, but the difficulties of achieving such changes are made evident in my discussions of many of the cultural interventions analysed in this volume.

From 'dying from' to 'living with' HIV/AIDS

The mourning which dominated representations of and theoretical analyses of works on HIV/AIDS in the late 1980s and early 1990s has, in some respects, receded in the late 1990s as changes in knowledge about HIV/AIDS and in treatment regimes, especially as practised in western countries,[16] have meant a move from a dominant notion of 'dying from' AIDS to 'living with' HIV/AIDS. Jackie Kay's poetry, discussed in Chapter 5, exemplifies that shift. In her 1991 collection of poetry entitled *The Adoption Papers* mourning dominates the poems directly concerned with HIV/AIDS. In her later collection *Off Colour* (1998) the tone is rather different. Still working on the relationship between race and colour, between what is visible and what is hidden, figurations of the body, illness and health, her poetry has moved to a repudiation of the preoccupation with the sick, different or marked body which seemed to dominate cultural thinking and representation in western culture at the turn of the millennium. We may think we are *dying from*, but, as Kay's later poetry suggests, we are in fact *living with* our bodies, whatever shape, colour, form, identities these take, and that, in a sense, despite rather than because of ourselves. Kay's *Off Colour* condenses various histories of epidemic to suggest that, whilst the body has remained marked as stricken by disease, it has in fact outlived epidemics such as the bubonic plague and continues to exist beyond the moment of marking. The rampaging, exuberant virus, personified in these poems, becomes the emblem of a surviving corporeality which defies the elegaic stance of Kay's earlier work, and HIV/AIDS cultural consciousness as it manifested itself in the early 1990s.

This version of a surviving corporeality stands in marked contrast to earlier representations of HIV/AIDS in which mourning and militancy were co-present as part of the attempt of making real the real of HIV/AIDS for those directly affected by it through its visibilization in films and on stage. Larry Kramer's theatre work is one such example. But, as I suggest in my discussion of his plays in Chapter 6, Kramer's return to the trauma of his expulsion from Gay Men's Health Crisis and his re-visiting of the family scene in *The Normal Heart* and *The Destiny of Me* resulted in representations of the real imbued with the norms and conventions of bourgeois theatre which confirmed the otherness of those suffering from AIDS-related diseases through their death and (thus) guaranteed the mainstreaming of his plays. The same might be said of *Philadelphia*, analysed in the Conclusion. In this film it is less the death from AIDS-related diseases of the protagonist which is mourned than the liberal state's difficulty in maintaining a just society while protecting 'us' from 'them'. The protagonist is constructed as deviant and devious, indeed devious *because* deviant; his ability to penetrate the inner sancta of elite society and the law through passing as seemingly heterosexual and healthy is exposed as a temporal performance which when discovered justifies banishment, easily accomplished through death. *Philadelphia* asserts that a certain truth, the logic of the real as constructed by mainstream society and made manifest through becoming visible (in this instance literally, through the lesions which appear on the protagonist's face), will out and that justice will be done within the conventions of that real.

The conventions of that real demand the perpetual othering of those perceived to be different. The film therefore carefully distinguishes between its gay protagonist, the devious and deviant one, and another person with AIDS, a Mrs Benedict, who acquired HIV through a blood transfusion. While the protagonist dies, she lives and represents the surviving corporeality referred to above in relation to Kay's poetry. *Philadelphia* thus points to one of the dilemmas which faced us in the late 1990s as both dying from and living with AIDS occur. The dominance of mourning which shaped interventions and responses to HIV/AIDS a few years ago has given way to a recognition that diversity is now the rule of the game, that many live with as well as die from AIDS, that disease patterns and infection patterns have become increasingly diverse, draining the energies from a concerted and unified effort to combat HIV/AIDS to a fragmentation and multiplicity of this effort which has made possible the re-invisibilization of HIV/AIDS. HIV/AIDS has acquired an everywhere-and-nowhere status which has re-domesticated HIV/AIDS, drawn it back into specific communities and into particular agendas which seem no longer to require coalitions and alliances. A gap has emerged which is concentrated less on the differences between the homosexual and heterosexual communities of the western and northern worlds, and much more on the division between south and north, between poor and rich. As indicated in Chapter 4 and in the Conclusion, the treatments now available to those who are more affluent in northern communities are not affordable for many southern countries, but the spatialization of HIV/AIDS across geographies mapped on to patterns of relative wealth and poverty has redrawn the boundaries from within which HIV/AIDS interventions occur, generating the (re)new(ed) invisibility of HIV/AIDS among dominant northern communities. Implicitly, this volume therefore charts, in a sense, two contrary movements: the rise of HIV/AIDS as a disease pattern and its fall in visibility in the social imaginary of contemporary western culture. Always already associated with the other, HIV/AIDS managed only briefly to transcend the boundaries of the visible world to enter the visual, cultural imagination as a signifier of catastrophe, and then under very specific conditions in which a sense of HIV/AIDS being about unprecedented numbers of deaths among gay men was dominant, and the threat of an over spill into the community at large seemed imminent. The seeming containment of both,[17] the one through education and prevention work, mainly done from

within the gay community, the other achieved only partially in northern and western communities[18] where the rise of infection and disease
among women, poor people and drug users continues to be ignored, has
displaced the anxieties which guaranteed the scripto-visual space for
HIV/AIDS intervention work. For many living in the UK and the USA,
and other western countries, HIV/AIDS has clearly withdrawn behind
an invisible boundary beyond which only the other resides.

Coda: issues of terminology

Throughout this volume I use 'HIV/AIDS' to encompass both reference
to the virus (human immunodeficiency virus) which, as Wilton (1997)
puts it, 'damages the immune system to such an extent that infected individuals eventually go on to develop AIDS (acquired immune deficiency
syndrome)' (xi), and reference to this syndrome. Through this compre-
hensiveness I hope to avoid some of the pitfalls of (mis)use of HIV/AIDS
terminology Watney (1989a) and others have critiqued.[19] Occasionally I
use the acronyms HIV and AIDS on their own, usually in a context that
makes clear why such usage is called for in the specific instance.

Notes

1 For a discussion of issues arising from HIV/AIDS (re)presentations in art see Chapter 3 of this volume.
2 As has been variously suggested, women play indeed a pre-eminent role in caring for
those with HIV/AIDS (see Gorna 1998; Roth and Fuller 1998).
3 I use the phrase 'lesbians and women' to point to an on-going debate about the concept of 'woman' and the notion of both 'lesbian' and 'woman' as construct. For further discussions see Wittig 1992; J. Butler 1992; Frye 1990; Radicalesbians 1970; De
Beauvoir 1949.
4 The notion that lesbians engage in nurturing long-term relationships whilst gay men
have a sexually promiscuous lifestyle has, of course, become contested, especially
since the rise of 'queer'.
5 A typical comment from the period was that if you went to a benefit organized
by and for gay men, tickets were £50 and it was a dressing-up affair, whilst benefits
organized by and for women or lesbians usually asked for 'bring-and-share' bags
of food. This is, of course, powerfully reminiscent of Virginia Woolf's account in *A
Room of One's Own* (1929) of the difference in wealth between women's and men's
colleges in Oxbridge, and this impact this has on women's cultural activity and social
status.
6 I return to this issue in Chapter 7.
7 Gorna (1997) raises the issue of 'AIDS envy' (350) as a reaction formation to lesbians'
perception that gay men swamped the lesbian and gay rights agenda with the
HIV/AIDS issue. She describes it, appropriately, as a 'hateful phrase' and I personally have yet to meet a lesbian who suffers from such envy.
8 *Derek Jarman's Garden* (1995), brilliantly photographed by Howard Sooley, is a striking testimony to this preoccupation and articulation of detail in Jarman's work.

9 For a very nuanced discussion of the uses of elegy in the context of HIV/AIDS see Woods (1992).

10 I use 'people' here despite agreeing with Watney (1997: 83-6) that that word obscures the realities of who is affected by HIV/AIDS and how. I do so not because I am interested in apportioning any kind of blame or singling out specific groups but in order to highlight a dilemma which, in my view, is faced by all those trying to seek representation in relation to HIV/AIDS.

11 Cancer has generated a whole range of important *textual* responses (see Lorde 1980 and Stacey 1997, for instance) but, perhaps with the exception of Jo Spence's work (1987; 1995), not nearly as powerfully in the visual field as HIV/AIDS has.

12 I write 'seemingly unprecedented' because, as many responses to HIV/AIDS showed, deathly epidemics involving the sudden loss of many lives have occurred before (see, for instance, Gilman 1988b; Fee and Fox 1988).

13 See for instance Juhasz 1995; Lupton 1994; Patton 1990.

14 I use 'objectifying' to denote the making of an object, not to suggest impersonality or the demeaning domination of an other.

15 *Bodies that Matter* was conceived in part, as its introduction shows, as a response to the criticisms levelled at Butler's ground-breaking work, *Gender Trouble*, of 1990. I shall not discuss here the debates about performativity raised through that dialogic exchange with her previous publication.

16 In Chapter 4 I discuss some of the issues related to the differential impact of HIV/AIDS in western countries and African countries where poverty, for instance, militates against the wide spread use of the expensive and difficult-to-administer combination treatments now available to those westerners who can afford them.

17 See Oppenheimer and Reckitt (1997) and UNAIDS/WHO (1998) for representations of the current state of affairs regarding numbers of people suffering from HIV/AIDS, the kinds of interventions required, and education and treatment issues.

18 As discussed in the Conclusion, UNAIDS/WHO (1998) presents depressing figures of the spread of HIV infection and occurrence of AIDS-related diseases in African countries, South Asia and East Asia.

19 In chapter 4 I briefly discuss the debate about the relationship between HIV and AIDS as it has taken place in medico-cultural contexts.

1

Visibility blue/s: Derek Jarman's *Blue*

> It sometimes seems as though everything in my past has been a kind of extended excuse for experiments with subject position and interaction. After all, what material is better to experiment with than one's self? (Stone 1996: 2)

> AIDS does not exist apart from the practices that conceptualize it, represent it, and respond to it. We know AIDS only in and through those practices. (Crimp 1991: 3)

It is 1993. Derek Jarman's film *Blue*, just released and even then already described as his last film – death foreshadowed – is touring the UK's alternative arts venues. I go to see it at my local arts cinema, one mid week evening, when it has been showing for a couple of nights already and has only two more days to go. I know little about it. But I – like the rest of the audience? – know that Jarman is gay and that he's dying from AIDS. The cinema is empty; I am the first to arrive. Not many more will come. A sign of the times? After the flurry of engagement with AIDS in the late 1980s and very early 1990s – as evidenced in the number of films, exhibitions and demonstrations which happened then – it seems that the mid-1990s are a period of silence, of absence, as far as AIDS is concerned. It does not have much of a presence in the media, the general public appears uninterested, unconcerned. Hence, perhaps, the very small number of viewers of *Blue* the night I go to see it.

Seeing *Blue*

Shortly after I arrive in the cinema, a group of four, two women, two men, students possibly from one of the two universities in the town in which I live, enter the auditorium with its fixed, tiered seating. After looking around briefly to decide where to sit one of them heads towards the second row from the front, followed by the others. As they thread their way towards their seats, the second man (jokingly as it turns out) asks the one who leads the group: 'Why are we sitting so close to the front? Are you afraid of missing any of the details? You'll certainly get a really good close-up view of everything from here.' Whisperings and laughter follow.

This, in a sense, is the beginning of this book because, as becomes evident when the film begins, there is *nothing* to see. That, at least, is the initial impression. A blue, blank screen confronts the viewer for all of the seventy-five minutes during which the film runs. The effect is extraordinary. The gaze, used to representational material on screen, meets a visual void in a context – cinema – where visuality is everything. In fact, it is perhaps not so much a blank as a lack of spatial depth that one encounters, a lack which prevents the eye, used to searching out differentiation, from fixing on such points.[1] I think of cinema, like the visual arts, as a visually over-determined medium, so to be confronted by a monochrome screen which does not change is very disconcerting.[2] Its minimalism takes you aback. It creates a disruption as the cinematically conditioned expectation of what one 'usually' sees on film at the cinema is not met. In the early stages of viewing the film I try to create differentiation on the undifferentiated surface, look for something my eye can focus on, the effect of a scratch on the camera's or projector's lens, for example, or something, anything for my eye to hold on to. There is an intense desire to *see*. In cinema we are *meant* to look and to see: we expect our gaze to be met by, or to meet, an object to behold, a moving, changing object at that. But, as Parveen Adams (1996) writes: 'The question of perception must take up the problem of what I want to see, and the way in which it structures the gaze which captures me. Instead of thinking of perception as just a visual field, it must be thought of as the field that is structured by relations and forces of objects and desires' (111). In *Blue* looking and seeing acquire new meanings because the gaze is denied, or rather the desire for the gaze to be met by a visual object is unexpectedly re-directed. For it is, in fact, not exactly the case that there is nothing to see – what we have is an immense, screen-filling blueness, and, as a gaze accustomed to representational painting needs to adjust to the abstract works of, say, Mark Rothko, so the viewer's gaze in *Blue* needs to adjust away from the representational expectations conventionally met in cinema to a non-representational, unchanging surface.[3] In this context and in this film, looking acquires – for me, at least – a meditative dimension, coupled with a re-focusing of the senses, away from the visual and to the auditory. As Michael O'Pray puts it: 'It is as if a cacophony of sounds has supplanted the pandemonium of images' (1996: 73). One of the film's gestures is thus that it in a sense asks one to listen. It also raises the question, to which I shall return below, of why listening – as opposed to viewing – is privileged here.

It takes some time for the film's voice-over, Derek Jarman's, John Quentin's, Nigel Terry's and Tilda Swinton's associative comments, meditations on the colour blue, and on Jarman's condition as someone in an advanced state of suffering from AIDS, to produce an effect which changes my relationship to the screen image, or its absence, for me to immerse myself in the colour I am offered and to start, like Jarman, to think about that colour, to develop, in parallel, sometimes overlapping, sometimes diverging, associative thoughts on blue and how these associative processes, the blue screen and Jarman's words on his condition intersect. It is an extraordinary and absorbing experience.

Militant acts of mourning

Jarman's *Blue* constitutes in some ways one of the 'personal, elegiac expressions that appear[ ] to dominate the art-world response to AIDS' as Douglas Crimp (1991: 15) puts it. In this respect it reflects both 'the new intersections between sexuality and death which AIDS has reintroduced into popular consciousness' (Altman 1994: 168) and the fact that cultural responses to AIDS 'grow[ ] out of the experiences of those most immediately affected' (Altman 1994: 167). As Jarman wrote in *At Your Own Risk*: 'The problem of so much of the writing about this epidemic is the absence of the author ... It is no good alerting the "public" while distancing yourself' (1993: 5). This links very closely with Jarman's experience of being gay as he describes it in his autobiographical writings where there was an absence of 'authors', of people who acknowledged their gayness in ways which enabled young homosexuals to feel at ease with themselves and their sexuality (e.g. *At Your Own Risk*, 1993: 37–8; *Modern Nature*, 1992: 58). Similarly, the experience of being one of the few men 'out' as HIV-positive cast Jarman into a particular position as outsider: 'It is a minefield to be one of the few identifiable HIV-positive men in the world, realising whatever I said might be taken as representative. My age, experience, work, were all different. The pressures of HIV are as numerous as the people who have to cope with them ... I never thought through what the HIV announcement would cost me' (1993: 123). Out of all these experiences, and not out of the blue, comes *Blue*.

One might argue with James Cary Parkes (1996) that 'Even before AIDS, gay art and the "homosexual sensibility" wore the weight of elegy. Melancholy and mourning are the poetic legacies of prosaic oppression and menace – this is not to say that the tradition of *outsider* existence is necessarily tragic or dour, but rather that a history of brutal and ethically unjust treatment endows a particular perspective on society' (138). The difficulty for Jarman was how to combine the personal with the political so as not to fall prey to sentimentalism, narcissism or an inverted homophobia whereby the representation of HIV/AIDS serves to reinforce the notion that it is the '*gay* plague'. As Douglas Crimp (1989a) stated: 'I think that there are very specific dangers inherent in art shows about AIDS' (8). Jarman himself was fully aware of these. In *Derek Jarman's Garden* he wrote: 'The garden was made into an AIDS-related film but AIDS was too vast a subject to "film". All the art failed. It was well-intentioned but decorative.' (91). Jarman was horrified by the sentimental, the decorative and the domestic in AIDS-related cultural production, all of which defies the purpose of activist art. He described himself as 'a passionate militant' (1993: 125) and, as such, he gave voice and image to a condition, the rise of HIV/AIDS, which shaped homosexual life and culture of the 1980s and 1990s.

Jarman's militancy is partly realized through his work as an artist and within that specifically through the simultaneous presentation of his own experiences and gay experience (if indeed there is such a unitary concept) in general. In *At Your Own Risk* he wrote: 'most of the works on our Queer lives underestimate the effect of art in favour of political action;[4] I think this is wrong. I know that my world at eighteen wasn't the gift of politicians but of the identifiable homos' (1993: 46). What needs to be distinguished between here, perhaps, is – as Tessa Boffin and Sunil Gupta (1990) put it – 'the difference ... between the politics of representation and the *representation of politics*' (1) or the politics of a particular representation as opposed to the representation of a particular politics. Jarman engaged both with the politics of representation and with the representation of politics (see Brabazon 1993).

In 'Mourning and militancy' Douglas Crimp (1989b) discusses the relationship between mourning (which may find artistic representation) and militancy (political intervention). As the paratactic title of Crimp's essay indicates, he regards mourning and militancy as two potentially opposing and/or mutually exclusive positions which need to be allowed to co-exist. Developing this I would argue that mourning can be militancy, that what Crimp reads as the description of a debilitating condition in Sigmund Freud's (1917) essay 'Mourning and Melancholia', namely the focusing down which is associated with mourning and melancholia, may in fact be the source of an enabling activism through the concentration of all energies on one issue.[5]

Visualizing mourning

Blue raises many questions. But the one I want to focus on and start with in this book is why HIV/AIDS, a visually under-determined illness, surfaced in cultural representation in visually over-determined media (film, theatre, photography, poster campaigns, art). As Edmund White (1994) writes: 'The most visible artistic expressions of AIDS have been movies, television dramas, and melodramas on stage' (132). *Blue*, through the particularity of its screen image, through its 'empty' screen, articulates this phenomenon especially powerfully and in a manner quite unlike any of the other visual 'texts' on HIV/AIDS.[6]

The 'emptiness' of the screen in *Blue* surfaces issues of visibility and invisibility. Jarman cinematizes an absence which the audience is invited to fill, aided by the sound track and voice-over which accompany the film. One narrative strand of the film's meditative commentary details Jarman's gradual loss of sight[7] and the effects this has on his interactions with his environment. Thus when he offers to share his taxi with a woman who has been to the same hospital as he has and she bursts into tears he finds, 'I am helpless as the tears flow. I can't see her. Just the sound of her sobbing.' Jarman enables the audience of *Blue* to share his experience of being unable to see – the helplessness derived from loss of vision. The audience's experience of seeing 'nothing' thus parallels Jarman's experience of sightlessness and creates a point of identification[8] between Jarman and the audience. This also reinforces the importance of vision as a medium for engaging with others – we need to be able to have, or make, an image of the world and other people around us in order to know what to do.

Jarman's text for *Blue*,[9] a diary of sorts of the progress of his illness ('My sight failed a little more in the night'), constitutes a raging[10] against the dying of the light in the face of the recognition that 'I shall not win the battle against the virus – in spite of slogans like "Living with AIDS" ... Awareness is heightened by this, but something else is lost. A sense of reality drowned in theatre / / Thinking blind, becoming blind' (Jarman 1993a: n.p.). Jarman's representation, however, is not one of panic. It is, rather, about the dailiness of dealing with AIDS and, specifically, about 'hav[ing] to come to terms with sightlessness' (1993a: n.p.). In his autobiographical texts, produced prior to *Blue*, Jarman expressed his fears concerning the effects of being HIV-positive on his mind and body: 'I worry about blindness and the degeneration of the mental faculties; I worry about the disfigurement of Kaposi's Sarcoma – one of my acquaintances had this when the virus was first isolated, and I'm ashamed to say I hardly dared look at him' (1993: 113).[11] In these writings, Jarman admits: 'I am vain. The thought of being disfigured by the illness seems to me more horrendous than the illness itself. Perhaps I would gain the courage to go out and realize it wasn't so devastating. I feel marked out as a public person with HIV' (1993: 116). Jarman's fear of losing his looks, his mourning for the physical changes to which his body is object and subject, is met in *Blue* by the absence of an image. Unlike the film *Silverlake Life: The View from Here* (1993)[12] which, as Phelan (1997) puts it, '[r]eversing the mainstream cultural imperative that constructs AIDS as shameful, humiliating, and obscene ... gives the dwindling materiality of the AIDS body an awesome ocular weight' (154), *Blue* does not present the viewer with a human body to behold; instead it both escapes, and returns us to, the experience of HIV/AIDS as a specific physiological occurence – it asks of the viewer, what do you expect to see?

Jarman does not use the documentary format to delineate *his* specific AIDS narrative (although it is simultaneously his autobiography and his art work); to do so would mean, *inter alia*, to chart the body's decline, to repeat the narrative of 'diagnosis to death', with a pre-HIV/AIDS golden age of sexual freedom possibly thrown in as a preamble. For Jarman, the man who fears his body's disfigurement through disease 'more than the illness itself', this would have been an actualization of a potential nightmare. In the film the mourning of the loss of the body beautiful is therefore achieved differently, through the creation of another body beautiful, the film.[13] This is particularly significant in a context where the representation of the dis-eased body has served to construct 'guilt by differentiation' as Tamsin Wilton puts it (1992: 27-31), in other words, where the person with AIDS 'usually hospitalized and physically debilitated, "withered, wrinkled, and loathsome of visage" ... is [presented as] the *spectacle* of AIDS, constituted in a regime of massively overdetermined images' (Watney 1991: 78). Watney (1990a) points out that this '"look" of AIDS faithfully duplicates previous ideas and fantasies' (182) about gay men rather than any 'truth' about the illness. He maintains that 'the ideological construction of AIDS as emblematic of otherness' (1989a: 19) has been promoted by heterosexist society and has encouraged those who do not have HIV/AIDS, particularly heterosexuals, to consider themselves as immune from the disease. HIV/AIDS has thus become another vehicle for expressing homophobia.

As Douglas Crimp (1991) and others have made clear, all HIV/AIDS representations reflect and feed particular political positions, one of the most prominent of which has been the presentation of the person living with HIV/AIDS as a victim, to be seen as other, ostracized and, in any event, near death, therefore at the end of a particular narrative line which is resolved through the AIDS victim's death. In *Blue* Jarman refuses this specific narrative. As Erica Carter points out: 'categories of "otherness" [are] occupied by the sick, the aberrant, the socially deviant' (1989: 62). The impact of this as regards representations of people living with AIDS is that by presenting such people as 'mute victim and vision of horror' (Carter 1989: 60), their otherness is sealed. It enables those who perceive themselves to represent 'the norm(al)' (i.e. those not living with HIV/AIDS) to dissociate themselves from that image. Instead of the recognition of the image as a vision of a potential future self, the image serves to affirm otherness and thus 'enter[s] an *already* homophobic, blame-oriented culture obsessed with particular types of closed narratives' (Williamson 1989: 79).[14] Watney highlights the ways in which such representations serve to undermine any identification with homosexuals, constructing gay men instead as 'other' in order to preserve the 'fragile stability of the heterosexual subject of vision' (1991: 79).

Idealization and identification

The acceptance of homosexuality, on the one hand, and the understanding that HIV/AIDS is not particular to a pre-specified community, on the other, demand that this otherness is repudiated through identification. Kaja Silverman argues that idealization is 'the single most powerful inducement for identification', that it is therefore a crucial political tool and that 'We consequently need aesthetic works which will make it possible for us to idealize, and, so, to identify with bodies we would otherwise repudiate' (1996: 2). In its non-representation of the body suffering from AIDS *Blue* constitutes such a work. Silverman goes on to state that the identification such art works should produce must conform to an externalizing logic, i.e. they must resist incorporation by the viewer, therefore demanding active idealization, in order to refuse the narcissistic impulses which underlie all visual engagement and which prompt the viewing subject into categorizing what she or he sees into same and other. The absence of a literal, visual representation of a body in *Blue* means that Jarman refuses to situate or contain the look directed at the screen, thereby activating the viewer into an interrogation of her or his visual expectations and, simultaneously, denying an easy categorization of what is seen into same and/or other. The ideal that is represented, the colour blue, responds to an externalizing rather than an incorporating logic. As Jarman writes in *Chroma*: 'For *Blue* there are no boundaries or solutions' (1994: 115). *Blue*'s primary associations in western culture are with the sky, itself an emblem of the infinite, of dis-embodiment and transcendence.[15] These associations challenge the groundedness and embodiedness of how we think of HIV/AIDS, an illness located in the body and conferring on the body an express temporality which the art work itself, intended to exist beyond the moment of its creation, seeks to belie.

Living death

In its unvarying presentation of the colour blue the film suggests a permanence that the narrative itself queries. The stability of the colour is thus set against the variability of the sound. Things do change; the blue is an illusion. It thus throws into sharp relief the narrative of change which the film articulates. But this change is not evolutionary, predictable, steady, evenly spaced. Its diverse pacing is recorded via the voices and sounds which accompany the film. Elegaic, poetic sequences which utilize the present tense, the tense of infinity, alternate with documentary, factual statements that disrupt the aesthetic intensity of the poetic sections with a realism which highlights the need to manage the everyday experience of living with HIV/AIDS by creating diverse positions from which to inhabit that experience.

The voice-over of *Blue* begins with the sentence 'You say to the boy open your eyes / When he opens his eyes and sees the light / You make him cry out. Saying / O *Blue* come forth / O *Blue* arise' (Jarman 1993a: n.p.). The 'you' addressed could be Jarman talking to himself, Jarman instructing an other (who may or may not be a gay man), an unknown viewer. Quite what or who is being evoked remains unclear. But as with the 'empty' screen, so with the use of the second person: the viewer is activated through the address which might also be directed at her or him. This demand for engagement constitutes part of Jarman's militancy and is quite unlike the construction of the viewer's position in many other films on AIDS which, in their quasi-documentary, realist style foster passivity and distantiation in the viewer. *Blue* ends with another reference to a you: 'I place a delphinium, *Blue*, upon your grave' (Jarman 1993a: n.p.). Who is being mourned here? The self, Derek Jarman, is still, on one level, surviving. But simultaneously that self has also experienced death. 'Didn't you know I died years ago with David and Terry, Howard, the two Pauls. This is my ghostly presence, my ghostly eye. "I had AIDS last year," I said with a smile and they looked at me as if I was treating their tragedy flippantly. "Oh yes, I had AIDS last year. Have you had it?" / / Now it doesn't matter when I die, for I have survived' (1992: 10). The feelings expressed here are not unlike those of survivors of the Holocaust who have to come to terms with feelings of guilt about having survived the Nazi pogrom and Nazi concentration camps.[16] There is a difficulty in celebrating one's survival when all one's friends are dying and when one's own survival is uncertain. *Blue* says quite clearly that 'I, too, will die' but it does so without assuming a position of total annihilation or despair. Instead Jarman chooses the soaring blue of infinity. He does not produce a triumphalist narrative of overcoming, though; rather, his narrative projects ambivalence and asks the viewer to position her or himself. *'Endings'*, as Parkes puts it, 'are, paradoxically, invariably eluded' (1996: 138). I am not sure that there is a paradox here; the production of an ending also signals the end against which, in a sense, Jarman is working.

The film mourns many losses, of which that of eyesight is just one. There are the deaths of others from HIV/AIDS ('The virus rages fierce. I have no friends now who are not dead or dying'), terrifying deaths which speak to the uncertainty which is 'the worst of the illness'. *How* will I die becomes more important than *when will I die* when death seems a certainty. But the physical decline of the body, the loss of control over it, is not necessarily accompanied by a loss of mental control. The fearful question, 'If I lose half my sight will my vision be halved?' is answered negatively. But the mind cannot control the body – in the battle between the mind and the body, the body wins. Hence the disembodied voice-over in the film. Hence also Jarman's statement at the beginning of the film, 'What need of so much news from abroad while all that concerns either life or death is all transacting and at work within me'. It is the body that we recognize – without its presence there is nothing. This explains the primacy of the somatic in our lives, why Thomas needed to see.[17] Silverman (1996) maintains that 'our experience of "self" is always circumscribed and derived from the body' (9). In *Blue* this is realized through the absence of a literal body for us to behold, thereby working against a tradition of imaging in relation to HIV/AIDS which has centred on the presentation of the body in decline, coupled with the sounds that provide a representation of the body in decline.

Refusing the image

By 1993, when the film first appeared, the general public had become very familiar with a range of images – stills, by and large, rather than moving images – of people with HIV/AIDS.[18] These images have been widely critiqued[19] for the ways in which they constructed people with HIV/AIDS as individuals, outsiders, socially and culturally marginalized figures, carriers of death and infection, destroyers of families, morally corrupt persons, homosexual, alien, bound to *die from* rather than *live with* HIV/AIDS. Jarman's film offers a critique of those images by refusing the image as such. As he states in the film: 'The image is the prison of the soul, your heredity, your education, your vices and aspirations, your qualities, your psychological world.' Image, as Jarman presents it, is constructed not as that which controls perceptions but as the object of a sovereign subjectivity, unrecognized as such, perhaps, by the beholder who (re)creates the image in his or her own image but dominated by self-projection none the less. We recognize what we have been taught to recognize; we see or visualize what we have been encouraged to see. This is so for the image-maker and for the viewer. It constitutes the social basis of communication. The cultural construction of people with HIV/AIDS as victims, as isolated and as socially marginalized is all part of the phenomenon which decrees that those who have illnesses associated with sexually transmitted diseases are socially unacceptable (Gilman 1988a; Treichler 1991; Watney 1987: 38–57; Wilton 1992: 19–48). By refusing to construct such an image, indeed *any* image, for us Jarman intervenes in the image-making around HIV/AIDS and highlights the subjectivity of our perceptions. When viewing his film, we are invited to see with the mind's eye, to determine and interrogate the images we ourselves make of people with HIV/AIDS.

> I have walked behind the sky.
> For what are you seeking?
> The fathomless blue of Bliss.
>
> To be an astronaut of the void, leave the comfortable house that imprisons you with reassurance.
>
> (Jarman 1993a: n.p.)

This comfortable house which imprisons us is the preconceived image which absolves us from engagement, from needing to interrogate our subjectivity and our projections. The images that we might associate with HIV/AIDS will be different for those living with HIV/AIDS, either themselves or in terms of people they know, and for those who have no direct knowledge of people with HIV/AIDS. As Michael Bronski, a gay activist, writes: 'AIDS is on your mind every time the telephone rings, every time a letter from a slightly distant friend arrives. In Boston, a city not very hard hit by the epidemic, I know of thirty men who have died or been diagnosed' (1989: 220).

In 'Representing AIDS' Simon Watney (1990a), who as a writer on AIDS and AIDS activist was greatly admired by Jarman, argues powerfully for the need of an AIDS aesthetic, one that is politically engaged and which registers the diversity of those affected by AIDS and of their experiences.[20] Jarman's work in itself represents such diversity, for his autobiographical writings are very different from *Blue* (1993c) in their engagement with HIV/AIDS. Jarman regarded the announcement of his HIV status as 'a political act': 'it was politics in the first person' (1993b: 121). The effect of the announcement was that 'strangers I [met] in the street all [looked] on me as "dead". I [had] to underline the fact that I [was] OK; but doing this [did]n't convince them' (1992: 232). Quoting Jarman in 1997, as I do here, means acknowledging his death; having to change all the verbs from the present tense to the past tense creates an awareness of the fact that Jarman was living with, living – in a sense – *his* death at the time of writing. The idea that being diagnosed as HIV-positive equals a death sentence[21] is so entrenched in current cultural thinking that Jarman records of those who asked him about his illness, 'As the years passed, I saw in the questioner's eyes the frustrations of coming to terms with life; are you still here? Some were brutally frank: "When are you going to die?"' (1993b: 10) The simultaneity of life and death, the paradox of it which is in part the paradox of the unpredictability of HIV/AIDS, demands the construction of complex images to portray the uncertainty, the 'postmodern' condition of HIV/AIDS (Weeks 1990).

HIV-positive

In *At Your Own Risk* Jarman describes the impact on himself of being diagnosed as HIV-positive, which initially meant enacting the preparations for his own death both through making an 'elegaic' film, *The Garden*, prompted by the expectation of his imminent death, and through sorting out his belongings: 'Two years ago,' he writes, 'I wound up my life, wrote a will, and gave all my writing to the film archive … I had a three week period when I put my affairs in order, or was it disorder?' (1992: 122) The expectation of his impending death 'dis-ordered' Jarman's life in that it suggested both the need for re-ordering his affairs *and* the creation of a new order, one determined by death. But Jarman's survival beyond the appointed period ('When I was diagnosed five years ago, I thought I would be around for two or three years; that's the time you were given; that changed' (1992: 122)) necessitated a change in position – continuing to live but with an expectation of death. Jarman writes: '*Death out of the blue is horrendous to those outside but it is perhaps easier to die this way than with the uncertain threat of HIV*' (1992: 112; author's own emphasis) Jarman's liminal position between life and death (potentially the situation of everyone but heightened through illness) translated itself into activity and activism: 'At this moment, it hasn't caught up with me because I've buried myself in work, a way of coping with my situation' (1992: 116).[22] One might describe such work, as indeed Jarman does through his use of the phrase 'burying myself', as another kind of death, a death which works against the uncertainties created by HIV/AIDS through the taking of control, doing it yourself, becoming agentic rather than remaining the 'victim' of the condition.

Another way of looking at it, however, would be not in terms of the effecting of one's own death but as a means of 'enact[ing] the difficult force of a grief which simultaneously mourns the lost object and ourselves' (Phelan 1997: 153). Phelan describes the film *Silverlake Life* as 'a new manifesto for a politically motivated talking cure' (1997: 155). Something like this could be said of Jarman's *Blue*. Jarman's political intent is beyond question. The phrase 'talking cure' has a negative and rather derogatory connotation in British English in that it is associated with a middle-class therapy culture which is viewed very ambivalently in the UK. However, Phelan's argument that diaristic AIDS films may have the function of enabling both their makers and their viewers to mourn death, both their own and that of others, is an important and apt one. Phelan maintains: 'It may well be that the movie camera's greatest technological achievement is that it can ease our dying. It allows us to see what our busy vital eyes are too blind to see, and what our closing eyes most fear losing as they cease to see' (1997: 161).

In *Blue* Jarman achieves an intervention in the conventions of imaging people living with AIDS which insists on seeing, or understanding, not equalling looking and beholding. The screen in this film does not show objects; its surface deflects rather than reflects. It deflects both from an object, a body for instance, we might expect to behold and from our own immediate reflection. It requires re-orientation of cinematic and of image-related expectations on the part of the viewer. Neither the expectation that the gaze should be met by an image nor the expectation to see someone dying from AIDS is met. The re-orientation, then, leads back to self, a self that is specularly 'free' to roam the surface of the screen but whose thought processes and reactions are 'fed' by the voice-overs the film presents.

'Remember: To be going and to have are not eternal – fight the fear that engenders the beginning, the middle and the end' (Jarman 1993a: n.p.). The construction of *Blue* as a diary-like narrative, bounded by a knowledge of the gradual decline of Jarman's physical capacities and the expectation of his eventual death (in itself the conventional narrative of birth, life and death and thus expressive of the pattern of beginning, middle and end he seeks to resist through *Blue*), complete with an unchanging screen, offers no boundaries or solutions to the question of what the image of the person with HIV/AIDS should be. When Jarman writes: 'How are we perceived, if we are perceived at all? For the most part we are invisible' (1993a: n.p.), the first person plural, 'we', remains unqualified and could refer to anybody who chooses to experience herself or himself as included in this formulation. The film could thus be read as presenting a critique of the invisibility of HIV/AIDS and of homosexuals. But the 'we' retains an ambiguity of meaning which the film as a whole constantly underscores.

Jarman identifies fear as the motivating factor in the construction of narratives which have a beginning, a middle and an end, a fear that is mirrored by the representation of HIV/AIDS in the world at large which suggests, or strives for, representations that guarantee the intelligibility of HIV/AIDS, its readability through the fixing of origins, carriers, treatments, predictions of process and prognoses. As Gever (1991) puts it: 'The containment of knowledge about AIDS within familiar structures functions as reassurance for those worried about a "disease" that seems out of control' (110). Jarman's film refuses such reassurance and readability. Thus there is no image, only a colour to see, into or on to which viewers may project what they wish. Structurally, the narrative which is offered – though vaguely moving towards a closure which is death, for Jarman the certainty at the end of his illness – moves associatively, drawing on diverse discursive traditions in short vignettes which include lyrical sections, reported direct and indirect speech, first and third person narratives, passages in the present and in the past tense, diary-style telegrammatic sentences detailing daily routines and chance encounters. Structurally as well as visually it thus mirrors Jarman's assertion: 'The worst of the illness is the uncertainty. I've played this scenario back and forth each hour of the day for the last six years' (Jarman 1993a: n.p.). Jarman does not state what the uncertainty is that he refers to, nor does he elaborate further on the 'scenario' he has been playing back and forth. The particular thus becomes de-specified. Uncertainty pervades everything –

how you get the illness, what form(s) it will take, what course it will take, if and when and how you will die. This uncertainty mirrors the current state of knowledge in respect of HIV/AIDS[25] which can provide plenty of general indications of what might happen, of how HIV/AIDS might have developed, etc. but no certainties.

Jarman's film – even as it focuses on the story of one man – therefore does not set up a single figure as an exemplum; instead, he is simultaneously individualized and universalized (he is both unique and like others in his experiences). The first word in the film is 'you', which may be a way of Jarman talking to himself, effecting a dissociation from and objectification of himself or it may be a direct address to a (un)known other, potentially the viewer. The viewer is certainly offered the possibility of identification with the addressee but this is not the only position available. Similarly, the film ends with the phrase 'I place a delphinium, *Blue*, upon your grave' (Jarman 1993a: n.p.). Whose grave? Who or what is the other here? The end (of the film) is the 'grave' but the planting of a flower, especially one as phallically structured as a delphinium which points to the sky, is also a gesture towards life beyond – beyond the grave, beyond death. Life and death remain integrated in this final sentence. The I, facing death, faces death literally here in the grave of the other. This other is a 'you' whose undefinibility raises questions about the identity alluded to. Is it the laying to rest of the film *Blue*? Does it imply the laying to rest of all others whose deaths are also an inevitability? Is it the preparation of a site for a burial? I ask this last question because to talk of somebody's grave may be to talk of their death but does not necessarily mean that they have already died. The history of designated burial places attests to that. A grave may not contain a body either because none has been laid to rest in it (yet) or because the body has risen. Both the stories of Lazarus and of Jesus are instructive here because, if one is to follow Phelan's (1997) argument that those ostracized by society experience a social death, what we have in films on HIV/AIDS is the cultural representation of the dying of those already dead, which in itself implies a prior resurrection or second coming or rising from the dead – whatever one might wish to call it. Jarman maintains that 'all art is concerned with death' (1992: 117) and, to return to Phelan (1997) for a moment, this is indeed so, if we consider that art freezes and thereby – in the process of making – annihilates the living into a still, makes the present into the past whose recoverability and its not being live depend on the very fact that it is past. Phelan describes this particularly in relation to cinema which, she maintains 'has a specifically curative appeal in relation to mourning' (1997: 156) but, as Jarman suggests, this notion can be extended to all art.

Blue personalizes and depersonalizes the representation of a person with AIDS; it refuses to construct the image as either specific or general but particular to one group of people. The boundaries which supposedly guarantee intelligibility are thus obscured – what we may hope to or expect to see, the contours of lisibility, are set *not* by the film but by the viewer and the context in which we view the film, the cinema or the home if we watch the video. The effect is to move the content from being *there*, i.e. from an elsewhere, into a *here*, *into the presence* which is the environment and subjectivity of the viewer. The viewer thus becomes the presence which guarantees and structures what is seen, encouraged by the film as text and as (non-)image. And yet *Blue* also conforms to a tradition in HIV/AIDS-related cultural production described by Paula Treichler (1991) when she writes:

> Whatever else it may be, AIDS is a story, or multiple stories, read to a surprising extent from a text that does not exist: the body of the male homosexual. It is a text people so want – need – to read that they have gone so far as to write it themselves. AIDS is a nexus where multiple meanings, stories, and discourses intersect and overlap, reinforce and subvert one another. Yet clearly this mysterious male homosexual text has figured centrally in generating what I call here an epidemic of signification. (42)

Treichler implicitly acknowledges the fear Jarman referred to which generates the desire for a progressively structured narrative with closure. She also aligns this narrative with the subjectivity of the story-maker. But set against the idea of a multiplicity of meanings and stories is the supposedly homogenized body of the male homosexual, a figure which is at once the figment of the anxious imagination and the reality of the image. Jarman refuses this image. Jarman does not construct the film either specifically for a homosexual audience or as instructing a heterosexual audience, for example, about the issue of how to view HIV/AIDS and persons suffering from it; there is no sense inherent in the film of a predefined audience in terms of sexual practices. This raises an interesting question about who the supposed or desired audience for the film is, or, to put it another way, what different audiences might derive from the film. For, as Altman (1994) states: '[AIDS] culture becomes a form of activism and demands to be judged on both criteria: most of the artists who are moved by AIDS are not content with just recording the impact of the epidemic; they wish also to have an immediate effect on how it is perceived and regulated' (167).

In *Blue* the mourning for a specific individual – pre-emptive almost, as Jarman is not dead at the point of making the film – and his physical decline are mapped on to other losses which include the losses of friends who died from AIDS. As Edmund White (1994) wrote: 'To have been oppressed in the 1950s, freed in the 1960s, exalted in the 1970s, and wiped out in the 1980s is a quick itinerary for a whole culture to follow. For we are witnessing not just the death of individuals but a menace to an entire culture' (136). The threat of AIDS to homosexual culture is clearly articulated here, but *Blue* does not take quite the same line as White on this. *Blue* ends ambivalently, with the planting of a flower, often a symbolic gesture of hope, but on a grave, also the signifier of an end(ing).

Notes

1 I am indebted to Andrew Stephenson for pointing this out to me.

2 This is all the more so since Jarman as an artist tended to work in intense visual detail, creating visual excess rather than its opposite.

3 For another reading of this unchanging surface see Schwenger 1996.

4 Douglas Crimp, for instance, wrote: 'The really important work being done is out in the culture, dealing with larger audiences; it's not on gallery walls' (1989a: 8).

5 Larry Kramer's *Reports from the Holocaust* (1995) provides a vivid example of this.

6 One need only compare the film to Jarman's own parallel painting series entitled *Queer* and *Evil Queen* in which complex multi-layered images are produced which combine text and colour explosions to indict the popular press's reporting on HIV/AIDS and vent his frustrations over the phenomenon of HIV/AIDS itself.

7 In April 1993 Jarman also produced a painting entitled *Sightless* which was made 'after [he] had been blind for several months. He painted the process of going blind by taking colour photographs of his retina and splattering them with paint, symbolizing those dots and splotches which had begun by interfering with his sight and which, by the end of his life, had totally obscured it' (Morgan 1996: 119). A reproduction of this painting can be found in Wollen (1996: 127).

8 This point of identification is important in terms of empathy. In *Reports from the Holocaust*, for instance, Larry Kramer (19995) again and again points to lack of empathy as one reason for the failure of people and governments to intervene in the HIV/AIDS crisis.

9 One version of the text can be found in Jarman's *Chroma*.

10 A similar raging is visible in Jaman's paintings following his HIV-positive diagnosis on 22 December 1986, especially in the *Queer* and in the *Evil Queen* series.

11 Jarman's expression of fear of disfigurement here contradicts Schwenger's (1996) notion that 'in a curious way he almost welcomes the loss of images' (419).

12 *Silverlake Life* is an edited video diary of Tom Joslin's life following his HIV-positive diagnosis. The diary is both a love letter to his lover of twenty-two years, Mark Massi, who died in 1992, eleven months after Tom, also of AIDS-related illnesses, and a 'political statement about the impact of AIDS on the material, familial, and cultural body' (Phelan 1997: 154).

13 In *Over Her Dead Body* Elizabeth Bronfen analyses the ways in which the representation and discussion of death in a variety of predominantly nineteenth-century texts (pictorial as well as verbal) serve both to point to death and to construct death

as other, thereby recuperating the space of the living for the author: '[representation] is both mastery over negation and grounded on negotiation' (1992: 27).

14 As examples of such closed narratives, Judith Williamson (1989) analyses the use of the conventions of Gothic horror and sentimentalism in the construction of people with HIV/AIDS as other.

15 In 'Into the blue' in *Chroma* Jarman offers a whole range of associations with and cultural investments in the colour blue.

16 There have been repeated comparisons between the treatment of homosexuals in the context of the HIV/AIDS epidemic, and of Jews and homosexuals under the Nazi regime (e.g. Kramer 1995; Watney 1991).

17 In an interesting chapter entitled 'Whole wounds: bodies at the vanishing point' Peggy Phelan (1997) examines the relationship of the body, seeing and believing in connection with Caravaggio's painting *The Incredulity of St Thomas*, a painting particularly poignant here because of Jarman's own interest in the figure of Caravaggio.

18 See, for example, Watney (1991) and also *Positive Lives* (1993), edited by Stephen Mayes and Lyndall Stein, for a discussion of such images.

19 See Crimp 1991; Watney 1991, 1987; Gilman 1988b.

20 I think Watney's (1990b) critique of Gilbert and George's *Art For AIDS* exhibition (1989) because it re-directed the public eye away from a community-based exhibition, *Bodies of Experience*, defeats his final position which is a plea for diversity.

21 This consititutes a variation of the slogan SILENCE = DEATH adopted by ACT UP, and discussed in the next chapter.

22 See Chapter 1 in Elizabeth Bronfen's *Over Her Dead Body* for an apposite discussion of how Sigmund Freud presented coping with death through work.

23 Wilton (1997) points out that 'the clinical diagnosis of AIDS is subject to continual redefinition' (xi).

2

AIDSdemographics – ACT UP and the art of intervention

Unless we fight for our lives, we shall die. (Kramer 1983; rpt 1994: 33)

AIDS has reverberations across the whole spectrum of cultural practices, and ... strategies against it must *always* take account of AIDS in its cultural dimension. (Carter and Watney 1989: vii)

You should have a practice in art that actually looks forward to a moment that will be different. (Mary Kelly interviewed by Monika Gagnon, *C Magazine* 1986 (10): 24)

Fighting invisibility

Derek Jarman's film *Blue*, discussed in the previous chapter, was in part a response to the ways in which HIV/AIDS was constructed in the years preceding his own illness and death from AIDS. The emergence of HIV/AIDS in western culture in the early 1980s was hatched amongst confusion and alarm, produced by the problematic of its seeming incurability, its virulence and its instant alignment with the gay community by medical and other bodies. Its effect was initially to generate denial, displacement and a studied indifference or avoidance amongst the general populace, western governments and their agencies, and many in the gay and lesbian community. However, voices from the gay community began early on to rail against these attitudes. Amongst the now best-known texts from this period are probably Larry Kramer's articles '1,112 and counting' and '2,339 and counting', both of 1983. These articles as well as many others, and like the texts generated by the medical community,[1] created a particular image of the HIV infection (Patton 1989). As Kramer wrote, 'There are now 1,112 cases of serious Acquired Immune Deficiency Syndrome. When we first became worried, there were only 41. In twenty-eight days, from January 13th to February 9th [1983], there were 164 new cases – and 73 more dead' (1994: 33) What was alarming were the rapidly rising numbers both of those infected with HIV and of those dying from AIDS. The two seemed to rise in tandem, and, from the co-ordinates of those identified as HIV-positive and the numbers of those dying from AIDS, a correlation was drawn between the two which suggested the inevitability of death following HIV infection unless some means of halting the epidemic was found rapidly.

Government apathy in the early years of the AIDS epidemic is now well documented.[2] It included the failure to inform the general public about what was happening, the failure to provide accurate information reflecting the current state of knowledge regarding HIV/AIDS, the failure to counter inaccurate reporting, and the failure to provide or utilize funds for relevant research on treatment and drugs in appropriate ways. In the United States Larry Kramer among many others tried to speak out against this situation (see 1994). In the UK in 1988, seven years into the epidemic, Simon Watney – in comparing the work of ACT UP (AIDS Coalition To Unleash Power) in New York and the United States with what was going on in the UK at the time – could still write about the UK: 'This all speaks of a level of public involvement and engagement which remains sadly absent in the United Kingdom, where AIDS has not yet been widely taken up as a political or cultural issue, in spite of the fact that the situation of people with AIDS here is in many ways as bad as that in the United States' (Watney 1989a: 12). And Tony Whitehead, founder of the Terrence Higgins Trust, the first voluntary AIDS organization in Britain, pointed out in the same volume that a 'well-intentioned but perhaps misguided complicity between charity and the statutory sector' had enabled 'the latter consistently to avoid the fundamental issues and demands raised by the British epidemic' (Whitehead 1989: 107).[3]

Precisely because of these absences, the emergence of the HIV/AIDS epidemic generated a need for representation, a need stimulated by the particular patterns that were constructed by medics, the media, the 'general public' in the western world and, to some extent, the gay communities of that world, from the medical evidence which was made public knowledge. This evidence, which began to be published in 1981, indicated anomalous cases of pneumocystis carinii pneumonia (PCP) and Kaposi's sarcoma (KS),[4] a skin cancer among young gay men: 'PCP and KS are rare conditions among young middle-class men, yet cases were showing up on both coasts [of the USA]' (Grover 1989b: 11). And: 'all of the first patients reported were gay' (Grover 1989b: 11). This conjunction, which, as subsequent findings have shown,[5] was in some respects purely coincidental,[6] resulted in the construction of HIV infection and AIDS as a 'gay disease' or 'gay plague', emblematized in its early naming as gay-related immune deficiency (GRID). But the presentation of the gay community as carriers and victims of HIV/AIDS[7] necessitated counter-presentations or a counter-representation, understood here in three ways as

- creating a presence or making manifest,
- imaging, and
- mandation.[8]

The emergence of HIV/AIDS demanded the recognition, in the first instance, that an epidemic was taking place at all, that those affected had a right to support and help, that research was needed to understand HIV/AIDS, that drugs and other treatments needed to be developed and were required to help those with HIV/AIDS, and that prevention and education policies and training had to be put into place. All this had to happen in the face of rapidly growing numbers of infected and dying people.

In this chapter I shall consider one particular response to the HIV/AIDS crisis from the second half of the 1980s in order to examine how it sought to impact on the visibility and lisibility of HIV/AIDS and those affected by it.[9] The response or intervention[10] concerns the work of New York ACT UP, documented in *AIDSdemographics* (Crimp and Rolston 1990). In the next chapter I shall then consider government-initiated health campaigns in the UK and in Europe, and art exhibitions focusing on HIV/AIDS. These three constitute very different arenas of representation, indicative of the diversity of agendas that manifested itself in the course of HIV/AIDS intervention developments. They also function as indexes of the difference and relation between 'the politics of representation and the *representation of politics*' as Tessa Boffin and Sunil Gupta (1990: 1) put it in that they address in particular and diverse ways, implicitly and explicitly, questions about the nature and content of representation, its producers, messages, targets, audiences and effects, and, in so doing, the specificities of the in/visibility of HIV/AIDS.

ACTing UP

The speed of the growth in numbers of HIV-infected gay men and of gay men dying from AIDS, and the lapidary responses of western governments and their agencies promoted the establishment of ACT UP in March 1987.[11] ACT UP's interventions in New York constitute the now perhaps most famous HIV/AIDS activism undertaken by the gay community,[12] itself an indication of their effective engagement with the mass media, their ability to create a presence or visibility. For, critical to the success of any campaigns against HIV/AIDS, both mainstream and initiated by marginalized groups,[13] has been the harnessing of the mass media to the purposes of that campaign in reaching a wide(r) audience. As Crimp and Rolston state: 'ACT UP's media savvy thus showed itself from the very beginning, as did our ability to influence coverage by visual means' (1990: 31).

The importance of this influence cannot be over-estimated and for the following reasons:

- its impact on achieving visibility for specific HIV/AIDs issues and people affected by them
- its significance in depicting and constructing communities and subjectivities
- the significance of the visual domain for reaching a wide and diverse range of audiences
- its potential for effecting change.

As Watney (1992) has stated: 'Most people around the world continue to see AIDS not by direct experience, but through sources such as newspapers and television. Hence the profound significance of visual imagery, as it largely determines most people's perceptions of *all* aspects of the epidemic, from health promotion to questions of discrimination, prejudice, care, treatment, and service provision' (8). The relation between direct experience and visual imagery is of course a complex one. Indeed, on the basis of research done in San Francisco and a survey conducted by Crane Publications among employers who had or had not employed people dying from AIDS, Jan Zita Grover (1989b) concludes: '*personal experience*, not media messages ..., makes the critical difference in changing people's beliefs and behavior' (15). However, as the case of Kimberly Bergalis – a woman infected with HIV by a health worker who in the wake of her HIV-positive diagnosis became part of a virulent homophobic media campaign – demonstrated,[14] experience may lead to change but not necessarily in a desirable direction. More positive support for Grover's view comes from the findings of the Health Education Authority in the UK which suggest that, despite awareness-raising campaigns about HIV/AIDS aimed at heterosexuals, 'The over-riding concern in the late 1980s was the apparent complacency of a sexually active heterosexual population that believed HIV and AIDS did not (and would not) affect them, but "belonged" to gay men and drug users' (Field, Wellings and McVey 1997: 7). Where gay men's use of condoms as a preventive measure against HIV/AIDS had to some extent changed during the 1980s,[15] resulting in a (very) gradual decline in the numbers of those newly infected with HIV,[16] the heterosexual population remained difficult to persuade of the importance of such a change in behaviour, even when specifically targeted on this matter (Field, Wellings and McVey 1997: 10). Despite the complexities of the relationship between visual media and their impact, the point made by Watney that most people know about HIV/AIDS via mass media and specifically visual media remains and, as the impact of ACT UP's work and some of the health promotion campaigns for instance demonstrate, the visual media are an important, perhaps *the* most important, domain in the fight against HIV/AIDS, simply because the mass media especially are accessed by such a wide audience.

The art of intervention

It is within this context that the line taken by Douglas Crimp, an AIDS activist and member New York's ACT UP, has to be understood: 'art *does* have the power to save lives, and it is this very power that must be recognized, fostered, and supported in every way posible' (1991: 7). ACT UP, a 'diverse, nonpartisan group united in anger and committed to direct action to end the AIDS crisis'[17] (Crimp and Rolston 1990: 13), was created to counter the 'murderous regime of silence and misinformation' (Crimp 1988: 12) of the US government in the face of AIDS and with the aim, in the first six months of its existence, to get 'drugs into bodies' (Crimp and Rolston 1990: 37). In *AIDSdemographics* Crimp and Rolston provide a vivid account of ACT UP and some of its major early campaigns.[18] It pinpoints the specificities of ACT UP's interventions, which were characterized by

- the notion that art can save lives if used in an attempt to effect social and political change
- an understanding that art has to reach beyond the confines of traditional art institutions to effect change
- the specific targeting of governmental institutions, agencies and representatives who are key organizations or people in decision-making processes affecting work on HIV/AIDS
- a (re-)definition of the gay community in terms of agency and citizenship
- a highly organized intervention strategy
- professionalism in intervention
- speed – the ability to react very quickly to public events and

circumstances – designed to surprise the slow-grinding government machines but also to be topical and up-to-date regarding public policies affecting HIV/AIDS-related concerns

● the creation of a presence of ACT UP through disruptions which – especially when arrests for civil disobedience resulted – generated media attention

● the production of objects (such as leaflets, banners, T-shirts, badges, posters, other art work) with site- and context-specific meanings which could, none the less, be reproduced to similar effect in other contexts

● the specificity and explicitness of ACT UP's demands which were based on meticulous research and a clear understanding of the politics around HIV/AIDS work.

In relation to this last point it should be noted that the book *AIDS-demographics* itself 'is intended as a demonstration, in both senses of the word. It is meant as direct action, putting the power of representation in the hands of as many people as possible. And it is presented as a do-it-yourself manual, showing how to make propaganda work in the fight against AIDS' (Crimp and Rolston 1990: 13). The activating intention behind the volume was an extension of ACT UP's demands for activism and activity. ACT UP was very clear about the need to create effective propaganda in order to generate the changes needed to improve the situation of those living with HIV/AIDS. As Crimp and Rolston put it: 'What counts in activist art is its propaganda effect' (1990: 15). The propaganda effect of its campaigns thus became the key driver for ACT UP's interventions. However, the notion of a 'propaganda effect' does not specify the nature of this effect, and not all of ACT UP's campaigns were equally successful. The STOP THE CHURCH campaign in December 1989, directed specifically at Cardinal O'Connor,[19] backfired somewhat since 'Media coverage was extensive, distorted, negative' (Crimp and Rolston 1990: 138) and the Catholic community experienced the intervention as a desecration of one of its sites of worship. Crimp and Rolston's conclusion, 'Perhaps most important, STOP THE CHURCH taught us the necessity of applying rigorous political analysis to our choice of targets, with the goal of productive change uppermost in our minds' (140) indicates the need to harness any propaganda effect to productive change, as well as the difficulties of negotiating diverse discourses within the public sphere.

When ACT UP started to operate, its interventions were unlike any HIV/AIDS interventions because, instead of just focusing on activating and targeting the gay community as the 'main victims' of the HIV/ AIDS crisis, it turned its attention outwards, towards those with the power to effect change in the government's apathetic response to the crisis through the key role they played from within the dominant institutional structures. ACT UP established a multiple agenda with three main aims:

- to create visibility and cohesion among 'the movement' working to change the social conditions which promoted HIV/AIDS (Crimp and Rolston 1990: 19–20)
- to confront the government in its various institutional and personal manifestations with demands designed to alleviate the situation regarding HIV/AIDS
- to generate AIDS awareness and provide education through explanation and advice to the general population.

Interventionist art – silence = death

ACT UP's work, the images and signs they produced, were thus informed by a political rather than an aesthetic programme;[20] theirs was an art seeking to confront, challenge and transform, and as such they took what Hal Foster describes as an 'instrumental view of culture' (1985: 142) in which ACT UP, as active producers of cultural signs, also sought to produce specific meanings of their works, their images, posters, flyers and handouts. To do this, they developed similar tactics across a range of campaigns, namely to produce images and/with slogans, in other words to join the visual and the verbal, in order to create a specific scripto-visual message. The image thus did not 'speak for itself' but, rather, was in a sense spoken for, through the word. The verbal statements made by the work thus became the site of subjective and ideological activity, generating a vocal presence.[21] The signature logo ACT UP adopted, 'SILENCE = DEATH printed in white Gill sanserif type underneath a pink triangle on a black background' (Figure 1; Crimp and Rolston 1990: 14), which came to 'signify AIDS activism to an entire community of people confronting the epidemic' (Crimp and Rolston 1990: 14) is the classic example of this tactic. In terms of representational strategy, it borrows from conceptual art.[22] The image and words spoke to, about and from the movement against the epidemic: *to* and *about* the movement in that they reflect a particular hidden gay history (that of the extermination of homosexuals in Nazi concentration camps)[23] and suggest, by implication and to all those who read it (hence also *from* the movement), that to be silent, as people were in response to the actrocities committed by the Nazis, means death, possibly of those remaining silent but certainly of those persecuted. Simultaneously this slogan is an injunction to all those who read it, including those outside the movement, to recognize that silence equals death, as the rising figures of people dying from AIDS in the 1980s and early 1990s showed. Finally, it constitutes an injunction to speak, to counteract the silence which promotes death. As such the logo addressed the government of the day as much as other people in and out of the movement.

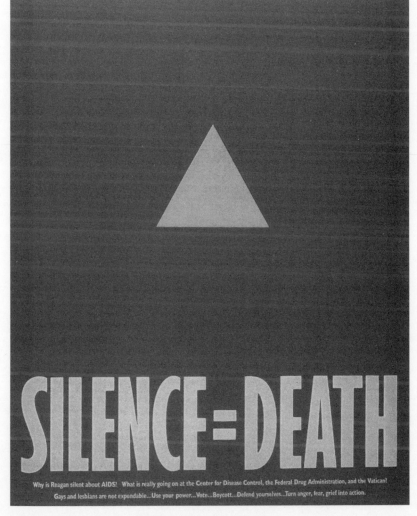

1 *Silence = Death* (1986)

The logo had seven key traits that are also specific to other ACT UP interventions:

1 it was simple and uncluttered, both as image and as text
2 it condensed a complex argument into a single message
3 it used quotation (of a historical sign) to make its point, thus giving it a wider context and culturally embedding it
4 it was easily reproducible and was reproduced
5 it was specific in its message
6 it arose out of collective endeavour
7 it was not created or owned by one particular person.[24]

It was the clarity, simplicity, condensation, reproducibility and specificity of the message which enabled it to become one of the key emblems of the anti-AIDS movement. The history which it betokened was a history of persecution.[25] However, importantly SILENCE = DEATH did not portray homosexuals as victims. The activism which led to the production of this image in itself constituted a counter-position to that notion. But additionally, its declaration that silence equals death enjoined its readers, gay and straight alike, to vacate that silence, not to allow another silence with all its historically well-documented effects to happen.

Since 'silence equals death' is equally significant for gays and straights, meaning that it as a position affects gays and straights alike in its assertion that one must speak out against injustice or risk death, the SILENCE = DEATH emblem was an important boundary breaker, disturbing the division between them and us, between gays and straights, in its injunction not to allow history to repeat itself. In this respect it was different from other images ACT UP produced as part of its campaigns where boundaries between 'them' and 'us', here defined as those refusing to work against AIDS as opposed to those who did, remained firmly drawn and were in fact used to shame the former.

ACT UP's interventions addressed three groups:

1 the gay community
2 the government, its agencies and agents, and the private sector (such as newspapers and pharmaceutical companies who stood to profit from AIDS)[26]
3 the non-gay populace.

I shall briefly discuss all three.

ACTING UP for the gay community

Stuart Marshall has commented on the importance of visibility in or through representation for the gay community: 'the visual domain has an extraordinary importance to gay politics and gay experience' (1990: 21). This is partly because, in a culture which relies on invisibility as a means of policing the assumed boundaries between 'them' and 'us', different kinds of visibilization become ways of simultaneously denying that difference and of identifying the different communities through signs related to, for example, appearance. Apart from the long history of visual markers (from specific colours to how and what things are worn) to signify homosexuality, Marshall highlights the significance of lesbian and gay presences achieved through the visibility of gay pride marches which function as a political tool: 'the Gay Pride march is the only political demonstration which automatically achieves its intended political end ... It demonstrates that lesbians and gay men exist, that we insist upon being visible and that we refuse to be confined to the private domain to which we have been consigned by law' (1990: 21). The usurpation of the public sphere by gays and lesbians both during Pride marches and in ACT UP campaigns for example, and public responses to these through the arrests of protesters, for instance, reveal the fallacy of the notion that in a democracy the public sphere constitutes 'a realm of free speech and open debate' (Foster 1985: 161). Instead, such actions index the illusion of unfettered access to the public sphere in a democracy, demonstrating that different groups exist in differential relations to that space, with some being allowed more access than others, and the display of certain discourses and sign systems being privileged within that sphere. Ironically, it thus plays into the hands of, for instance, the ACT UP campaigners by on the one hand generating visual over-determinacy when groups not normally visible in the public sphere decide to enter it, and reinforcing what ACT UP's images, *inter alia*, tried to suggest anyway, namely that public discourses on topics such as HIV/AIDS are partial in every sense of that word.

This partiality promoted the need for a counter-visibility and for (political) representation, both to support gays and lesbians through the so-called AIDS crisis and in order to counteract misinformation and indifference. ACT UP's interventions directed at the gay community were incitements to united action fuelled by references to gay and lesbian history which pointed to the destruction of homosexuals in the past as well as to the ways in which change had been brought about through action. A good example of the latter is the emblem (Figure 2) created by ACT UP for their Stonewall 20 march (Crimp and Rolston 1990: 98–107). The crack-and-peel sticker set the black header STONEWALL '69 against the red footer AIDS CRISIS '89, inciting the

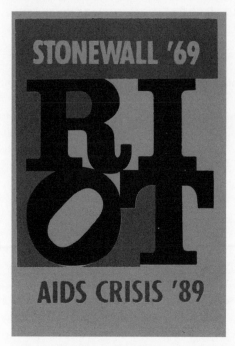

2 *Riot* (1989)

reader in the middle to 'RIOT'. As Crimp and Rolston describe it: 'The linkage STONEWALL '69 and AIDS CRISIS '89 by the exhortation to RIOT fit precisely with ACT UP's IN THE TRADITION theme' (1990: 102). Addressing a history of persecution but also a particular historical incident that ultimately ended in victory for the gay community, specifically because of the media attention Stonewall attracted through the act of rioting, this emblem references, and incites through, a notion of continuity and tradition which portrays the gay community as active and activist, and able to achieve its ends.[27] The inherently affirmative stance taken in this emblem is also evident in other visual signs created by ACT UP for the gay community. ACT UP thus produced and circulated images of the gay community which directly countermanded the imaging of that community in the mass media as victims. In so doing it projected the image of a collectivity rather than of individuals, addressing a community. This move is described by Foster as one effective way of creating disruption (1985: 176–8), partly because it refrains from personalizing or individualizing the issues. For, as Watney (1990b) puts it: 'By being repeatedly individualized, AIDS is subtly and efficiently de-politicized' (187). Instead, in the ACT UP campaigns addressing the gay community, the non-specificity of those

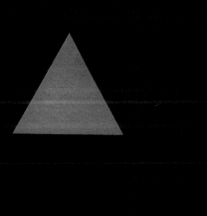

SILENCE = DEATH

Why is Reagan silent about AIDS? What is really going on at the Center for Disease Control, the Federal Drug Administration, and the Vatican? Gays and lesbians are not expendable...Use your power...Vote...Boycott...Defend yourselves...Turn anger, fear, grief into action.

1 *Silence = Death* (1986)

2 *Riot* (1989)

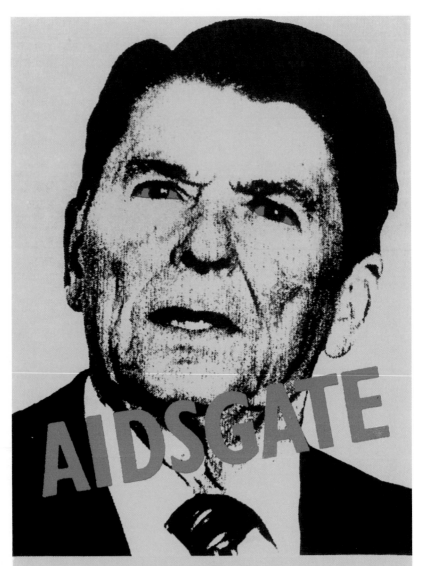

This Political Scandal Must Be Investigated!

54% of people with AIDS in NYC are Black or Hispanic... AIDS is the No. 1 killer of women between the ages of 24 and 29 in NYC...
By 1991, more people will have died of AIDS than in the *entire* Vietnam War... What is Reagan's *real* policy on AIDS?
Genocide of all Non-whites, Non-males, and Non-heterosexuals?...
SILENCE = DEATH

3 *AIDSgate* (1987)

who are gay created a counter-discourse to hegemonic versions of '*the gay man*', thus refusing type-casting: 'as [the media] transform[ ] people with AIDS into "AIDS victims," they themselves are actively contesting and resisting the discursive structures which they have been made to embody' (Watney 1990b: 183).

Confronting public inaction

ACT UP's address to the gay community was quite different from how it dealt with the government, its agents and agencies, and the private sector. Here many campaigns took as their object specific individuals or institutions who were directly asked to account for themselves and their (in)actions.Thus *The New York Times*, Wall Street, President Ronald Reagan, the Food and Drug Administration (FDA) and Cardinal O'Connor among many others were directly targeted.[28] Where the address to the collectivity of the gay community discussed above was intended to unite and generate strength and political power, here the highlighting of the specificity of individuals and institutions served to expose and disempower through accusation. Simultaneously, the singling out of specific individuals and institutions reinforced the historical, contextual specificity of the issues raised through representations with a politics. ACT UP's work sought to engage with the real in the sense of the social, cultural, economic and political realities it faced in order to create change within that real, a change that would impact on how HIV/AIDS was dealt with and on how HIV/AIDS was experienced. ACT UP located the possibilities for creating that change in those whom in its campaigns it showed up as responsible for policies and (in)actions which disenfranchised, and discriminated against, those constructed by the dominant discourse as suffering from or being responsible for HIV/AIDS. In each campaign which singled out specific institutions or individuals for attack, a context-specific image and text was produced (as posters, handouts, placards and in other forms), pinpointing the culprit(s) and his, or their, inactivity. In attacking these specific individuals and institutions ACT UP created a reverse discourse to the dominant one propagated by the media which made gays responsible for AIDS (Watney 1990b: 178). Responsibility was thus re-distributed to those who were in a position to intervene but failed to do so.

In each instance the preciseness and specificity of the campaign highlighted the particular demand that was being made, whether this be for 'Humane Housing for People with AIDS' (Crimp and Rolston 1990: 126) or as an indictment of '*The New York Times* AIDS Reporting is Out Of Order' (Crimp and Rolston 1990: 113). The imaging which resulted directed its beams not at gays but at the government, its institutions, agencies and figureheads as well as important non-government organizations such as the Church, which could have supported preventive AIDS interventions but failed to do so. Much of this publicity was accompanied by flyers and leaflets as well as on-poster or placard messages which reproduced facts about the AIDS crisis, researched by ACT UP. The fliers and handouts could be taken away from the site of the intervention, thus literally spreading the word.[29] Statements like 'US spends more in 5 hours on defense than in 5 years on healthcare' and 'NYC public hospitals: 37% of AIDS cases no money, no beds, no staff, no treatment' or 'NY State: 1982–1989 / Queer bashing triples' (Crimp and Rolston 1990: 106, 107, 105) confronted the viewer with material realities which demanded, by their very starkness and unflinching assertiveness, that they be engaged with. Written in the indicative, brief and simple, frequently supported by statistics, they detailed a state of affairs which condemned all those not working against the AIDS crisis.

Specifying the message

Central to ACT UP's campaigns was the integration of the pictoral and the verbal in a visual space. This contrasts significantly with most of the work produced for a mainstream art context, as discussed in the next chapter. In ACT UP's interventions the message was literally spelled out, not left to chance or the interpretive facilities of the viewer. A portrait of President Reagan is a portrait of President Reagan until and unless some other message is specified. ACT UP's work used words as part of an image, construction or installation to narrow down, thus make specific and explicit, the message and meanings it sought to convey. In this respect interventionist activist art was not about the ambiguity of meaning or polysemy associated with postmodern sensibilities, its task was not to activate the viewer to puzzle out semantic specificities – rather, the viewer was to be activated to, minimally, a revision of her or his views and, more promisingly in terms of effecting change, to further interventionist actions arising out of a greater understanding of how the government, its agents and agencies, as well as the private sector operate to create the deficits, inefficiencies, inaction and distress that dominated public responses to HIV/AIDS. In fact, for the purposes of ACT UP's activism, the primacy of the word as a visually placed agent becomes obvious. The words which form part of, or are, their images are the key to the significance of the image. In the hierarchy of signification, the verbal supersedes the visual to specify the meaning of the image. The logocentricity of hegemonic discourses is thus replicated and the latter are engaged with on their own territory.[30] As Griselda Pollock (1988) puts it: 'a strategic artistic practice ... does not operate from some imagined point outside the dominant culture. As practice it seeks to contest the hegemony of the dominant culture(s) by intervening in the relevant territories of production and consumption' (171). However, citing Roland Barthes, Foster (1985) has problematized the effectivity of such interventions by pointing to the ways in which 'criticism *within* the institution' and 'criticism *of* the institution' (158) may be subject to recuperation through '*innoculation*, whereby the other is absorbed only to the degree that it may be rendered innocuous; and *incorporation*, whereby the other is rendered incorporeal by means of its representation (here representation acts as a substitute for active presence, naming is disavowing)' (166).[31] However, what militates against both 'innoculation' and incorporation in this instance is the relative instability as well as the repetition of interventionist actions *per se* and the diverse targets ACT UP addressed, as much as the indeterminacy of HIV/AIDS, that is the difficulty of specifying its symptoms comprehensively, being able to categorize those affected by it precisely, and being able to particularize its progress. One might, of course, argue that the – albeit limited – responses to the demands of ACT UP and others for action against HIV/AIDS are an indication of an innoculation effect. However, since ACT UP as an organization was not rendered innocuous by these responses, this hardly applies.

Through filling silences with their words ACT UP intervened in the hegemonic discourses around HIV/AIDS which did not speak to or about certain conditions. Making the words manifest, embodying them in images, became a way of breaking the silence, of making the invisible visible. Through their images ACT UP constituted their members, those depicted and the spectators of their interventions as political subjects, suggesting a set of relations between them. These relations were predicated upon notions of activity on the part of ACT UP and inactivity or wrongful activity on the part of government oganizations and their agents. The images demanded that the spectator should position herself or himself in relation to the two. They also – through their accusations and demands – highlighted the disjuncture between the politicized subjects on the one hand and the government and the private sector in their various manifestations on the other.

ACT UP's campaigns thus made simultaneous statements about AIDS activists and about those indicted by the campaigns. AIDS activists were presented as well informed and knowledgable, competent tacticians in matters of disruption and civil disobedience, single-minded and outwardly focused. In contrast those indicted by the campaigns were revealed as incompetent, inactive or active through inaction, misinformed or uninformed, irresponsible, bigoted, and, often, murderous in their intent. This is evident in ACT UP's AIDSgate posters (Figure 3), which – underneath a Warhol-like image of Ronald Reagan's face – state: 'This Political Scandal Must Be Investigated! 54% of people

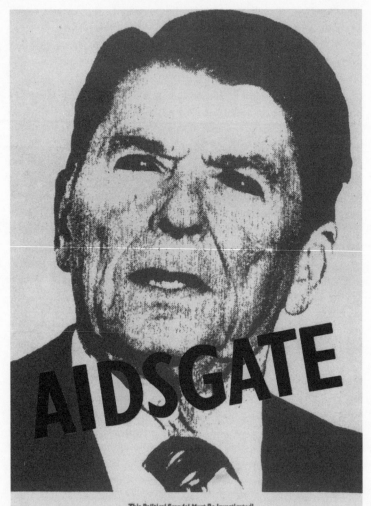

This Political Scandal Must Be Investigated!
54% of people with AIDS in NYC are Black or Hispanic... AIDS is the No. 1 killer of women between the ages of 24 and 29 in NYC...
By 1991, more people will have died of AIDS than in the *entire* Vietnam War...What is Reagan's *real* policy on AIDS?
Genocide of all Non-whites, Non-males, and Non-heterosexuals?...
SILENCE = DEATH

3 *AIDSgate* (1987)

with AIDS in NYC are Black or Hispanic ... AIDS is the No. 1 killer of women between the ages of 24 and 29 in NYC ... By 1991, more people will have died of AIDS than in the *entire* Vietnam War ... What is Reagan's *real* policy on AIDS? Genocide of all Non-whites, Non-males, and Non-heterosexuals? ... SILENCE = DEATH' (Crimp and Rolston 1990: 36). Here key statistics were combined with a demand for an investigation of Reagan's AIDS policy which suggested a policy of genocide and simultaneously, by pointing out those groups who would be affected by this policy. These groups, already victims of the government's non-intervention, as well as all viewers were incited to rise and protest against their own extermination. The truth which the statistics underwrite was spelt out in its implications in unambiguous terms, its meanings explicit. Watney (1997) has analysed the problematic of the use of statistics in official discourses on HIV/AIDS. ACT UP was creating a reverse discourse, utilizing the language and rhetorical strategies employed by public institutions, in order to highlight their inaction.

Breaking down the boundaries between 'them' and 'us'

ACT UP focused a number of campaigns neither on the government or private sector, nor on the gay community directly, but on either the population at large or specific sub-groups within the general population. Of these campaigns, several were designed to undercut the 'them-and-us' rhetoric which had informed campaigns like the takeover of the headquarters (see Crimp and Rolston 1990: 76–83). For this intervention ACT UP's Majority Actions Committee made a reproducible design for T-shirts and posters with the headline 'WE DIE – THEY DO NOTHING', detailing who was meant by 'we' and 'they'. The campaigns which obliterated that boundary aimed, in the main, to educate their viewers about the HIV/AIDS situation. One of the first of these was a sticker produced in 1988 by Little Elvis, an ACT UP collective, which stated, 'THE AIDS CRISIS IS NOT OVER' (Crimp and Rolston 1990: 43). Maintained against *The New York Times'* stance that AIDS was not a problem for anyone other than the gay community, THE AIDS CRISIS IS NOT OVER used the wasp colours of black print on a yellow background, conventionally one sign of danger but also associated with death, disease and contamination, to deny any suggestion that HIV/AIDS need no longer be taken seriously. This clever combination of colours and condensed message made the image instantly assimilable. The message, written in the indicative and using the tense of both the immediate and infinitute, the present tense, suggested truth and ahistoricity, thus defying the notion of a disease confined to those directly affected. It pointed to a ubiquity which *The New York Times*, for instance, was seeking to decry. The same principle informed the 1988 Gran Fury poster for the Spring Action which had the headline, 'ALL PEOPLE WITH AIDS ARE INNOCENT' (Crimp and Rolston 1990: 54–5). Again, the message was conveyed through words, a text that was integral to the image and which, since it was in the indicative and the present tense, confronted the viewer with a bold statement which both gestured to a citational chain within which it was situated and pointed beyond it by denying the historically specific. The citational chain of which some viewers at least would have been aware was, for the past as much as the future, the differential treatment given to, and perception of, different people with HIV/AIDS.[32] In late February 1999, for example, a debate occurred in the British media about the differential levels of funding on HIV/AIDS prevention work targeted by the health service at gay men as opposed to drug users, with the point being made that gay men, who constitute the highest risk group, get significantly less funding targeted at them than drug users.[33]

The citational chain of difference, established from the beginnings of the AIDS crisis through the epidemiological imperative to differentiate between so-called risk groups and supposed non-risk groups, coupled with the understanding of difference as inequality, generated the need – as the indeterminacy of HIV/AIDS unfolded – to counter-image the notion that only gay men were affected by HIV/AIDS and 'deserved' this, and that others need do nothing (other, possibly, than avoid gays) to protect themselves. The message from ACT UP was clear: such a stance was utterly untenable. They thus took it upon themselves, in a full understanding of the irony of this, to educate men *in general* and not just gays about HIV infection. As part of the nine days of nationwide AIDS-related activities and protests in the USA organized for 29 April to 7 May 1988 Gran Fury produced a poster aimed at heterosexual men (Figure 4), featuring an erect penis and the lines, 'SEXISM REARS ITS UNPROTECTED HEAD', 'MEN: Use Condoms Or Beat It', and 'AIDS KILLS WOMEN' (Crimp and Rolston 1990: 63). Going to sites where men rather than women congregate, ACT UP went to a ball game to unfurl banners about HIV/AIDS and to hand out fliers with a score card which stated:

SINGLE   Only *one* woman has been included in government-sponsored tests for new drugs on AIDS.

DOUBLE   Women diagnosed with AIDS die *twice* as fast as men.

TRIPLE   The number of women with AIDS *tripled* as a result of sexual

4 *Sexism rears its unprotected head* (1988)

contact with men in New York City since the 1984 World
Series.

THE
GRAND   Most men *still* don't use condoms.
SLAM

(Crimp and Rolston 1990: 65)

If one asks oneself, what would this have meant to the average heterosexual man (if there is such a man) in the conservative late 1980s,
one wonders how much they would actually have cared. Given the history of misogyny in western culture, and the conventional treatment of
women as objects and abject, I think heterosexual men might have
taken more note if the campaign had pointed at *their*, rather than
women's, vulnerability, simply because in my view women's vulnerability and hence, effectively, dispensibility is still very much taken for
granted in this society. Therefore the image presented on the score
card, to which men were I assume meant to respond simply because it
was a score card, presented something recognizably 'of-the-male', reinforced what is the normative view of women anyway.

In contrasting ACT UP's work with the history of Gay Men's Health
Crisis (GMHC), Stanley Aronowitz (1995) attributes ACT UP's success
in generating effective interventions and resisting incorporation into
the contract state through becoming a service rather than a campaigning organization to

- *the specificity of its organizational structure* in which 'control over
  ACT UP's policy is displaced from a putative center occupied by a
  swollen bureaucracy to autonomous voluntary committees which frequently vigorously disagree with each other, but are unable to veto
  the proposals of those with whom they disagree' (370)
- *the nature of its interventions* in which 'publicity is the movement's
  crucial strategic weapon, embarrassment its major tactic' (364) as it
  challenges 'the *ethical* legitimacy of the majority' (362), opting out
  of the 'vagaries of the procedurality of the liberal state' (365) and
  engaging in 'the politics of *terror*' (365) through refusing the trans-
  formation from adversary to collaborator as GMHC did
- *its understanding of postmodern politics* with its 'partial breakdown
  of the legitimacy of the liberal state' (360) in which 'the indeterminacy of the relation between electoral outcomes and public policy'
  (362) means that democracy's demands that 'citizens should be loyal
  to repressive civilization' (375) become a way of immobilizing these
  citizens, and in which those who show 'disrespect' for this demand
  can – by virtue of their disrespect – flourish.

Part of the disrespect resides in the publicity achieved through inter-ventions which attract media attention, thus reaching a wide audience who are involuntarily exposed to ACT UP's messages. As Aronowitz puts it: 'Rather than being fought *primarily* at the ballot box which in the eyes of most activists is stuffed by the de facto one-party system, the battle must be joined in the new public sphere: the visual images emanating from TV's 11 o'clock news of intransigent protesters con-ducting in-your-face politics, street actions that embarrass public offi-cials through exposure and other disruptions' (364). The importance of the taking-up by the media of interventions to combat HIV/AIDS is highlighted in Crimp and Rolston (1990) in accounts which point to the failure of the media to do so (e.g. 109–10). This represents an opportunity to publicize lost. Aronowitz also details, as do Crimp and Rolston, the successes of ACT UP generated through effective and widespread media coverage.

Active and passive subjects

ACT UP's activities did not go without criticism. A highly sophisticated one from Lee Edelman (1993) centres on the question of constructions of subjectivity in the face of HIV/AIDS functioning as an unmanage-able sign in Western culture, unmanageable because its meanings keep shifting. Edelman claims that 'the overlapping crises that we experi-ence as "AIDS" produce an oppositional discourse that has the poten-tial ... to naturalize and reposition certain aspects of the ideological structures that inform and produce those noxious representations and oppressive subjectivities in the first place' (13). Central to this opposi-tional discourse is the difference between the rhetoric of AIDS activism which assumes one kind of subject position on the part of the activist, that of agency, subject stability and 'truth' and the reprimands activist rhetoric explicitly or implicitly deals out to those who remain passive and do nothing, another kind of subject (or is it object?) position. Edel-man argues that in the history of cultural struggles about identity, 'only *against* women and gay men may the "normal male subject" imagine himself to *be a subject* at all' (22). This differentiation depends, *inter alia*, on the association between gay men and passivity, as emblema-tized in HIV/AIDS representations which associate AIDS with anal sex and its concomitant, the passivity of the man who 'is fucked'. Placing AIDS in its postmodern context and invoking the 'death of the subject' as one of the latter's paradigms, Edelman suggests that AIDS dis-courses, in their evocation of anal sex as a source of disease, reflect the notion of the death of the subject in three ways:

1 by projecting the symbolic death of the heterosexual male in favour of the homosexual male

2 by suggesting the death of the subject through the passivity of the man who is penetrated during anal sex

3 by conjoining the practice of anal sex with HIV infection and its supposedly inevitable correlate, death from AIDS.

In disputing these associations through their activism, AIDS activists recover the subject position and agency heterosexual men claim for themselves and, Edelman suggests, effectively '"our" "activist" discourse is only a *mutation* of "their" "master discourses" and that its effect on them, though certain, is also always unpredictable' (29). The 'political investment in a shared ideology of the subject' (25) between heterosexual men and gay AIDS activists which Edelman sees emerging here emulates, according to Edelman, 'the widespread heterosexual contempt for the image of a gay sexuality represented as passive and narcissistic' (27). Edelman views this as the 'internalization of dominant logic' (34), and argues that whilst activism is 'saving our lives' it need not do so by defining itself 'against the "narcissism" and "passivity" that figure the place of gay male sexuality in the Western cultural imaginary' (34).

Edelman's position depends on the construction of binaries such as active/passive, heterosexual/homosexual, activist/non-activist which replicate the dichotomous logic he considers to be inherent in western dominant discourse. The very fact, however, that he can point to differences among gay men (for example, activist and non-activist groups), and, indeed, that anal sex involves an active as well as a passive partner, already suggests the problematic of arguing within a dualist framework. Edelman does not critique this dualist framework; rather, he suggests that the disavowed term (passivity) might in time come to the aid of avowed one (activity) as '[a] necessary instrument of defense' (34). Edelman himself seems to believe in the notion of a unified subject since he regards the activism which kicks out at those in the gay community who remain inactive as a 'repudiation of all that "homosexuality" signifies historically in the West' (34). In a related footnote he indicates that he is not talking in essential terms but is pointing to a history of stigmatizing signification. However, and against that position, it has to be noted that activity (for example through the seduction of impressionable youths; through the notion of cruising) has also been a stigmatizing attribute in relation to the gay community. The binary framework which underlies Edelman's argument thus simplifies the pluralism, complexity and contradictions which inform the systems of signification within which we all operate and within which AIDS activism takes place. Edelman fears the incorporation of AIDS activism into the mainstream logic and representation of contemporary western culture; Aronowitz celebrates their defiance in the realm of politics.

There can be no doubt that ACT UP's work has been of major importance in raising HIV/AIDS awareness and achieving some changes in government attitudes towards and provisions for those affected by HIV/AIDS. In 1999 there were many chapters of ACT UP, and not just in the USA. Their early professionalism in their political work has translated into extremely well organized structures within ACT UP and effective interventions outside. This is reflected in the information sites they maintain on the Worldwide Web which detail both their continuing actions and their on-going research on HIV/AIDS. Their effectiveness, as the next chapter will indicate, has not been matched by that of either public health promotion campaigns or 'high' art, both of which also had the intention of making a difference.

Notes

1 See, for example, Treichler 1988; Gilman 1988a; Grover 1989b.

2 For an ironic summary, see Scott (1997: 307–10).

3 See Chapter 5, where the parallel problematic in relation to GMHC, the American Gay Men's Health Crisis organization which Larry Kramer helped found, is discussed.

4 For a discussion of KS see Knutson 1996.

5 As discussed in Chapter 3, the attempt to 'pin' AIDS to diverse specific communities at different times was predicated upon a perceived need to give the disease an identity and point of identification which would function as a boundary between those likely to be(come) infected and those unlikely to contract HIV. As is clear today, anybody can in fact become infected.

6 It is worth considering how issues such as body consciousness in the gay community, differential use by different communities of STD clinics, and access to health care provision in general influenced the picture of HIV infection patterns which was constructed in the early days of the AIDS epidemic.

7 See Watney 1990a and Grover 1989b.

8 Mandation here comes from 'mandate' and refers to 'the sanction held to be given by the electors to an elected body, to act according to its declared policies, election manifesto, etc.' (*Chambers 20th Century Dictonary*, ed. E. M. Kirkpatrick, Edinburgh, Chambers, 1983).

9 Everybody is, of course, either directly or indirectly, affected by HIV/AIDS. However, the history of health promotion exercises shows the ways in which different communities (whether imaginary or real) are constructed as being differentially affected (Field, Wellings and McVey 1997).

10 There is a difficulty with using either 'response' or 'intervention' here. The discussion about notions of passivity (= response) and activity (= intervention) in relation to HIV/AIDS work has been marked by its significance for the construction of the gay community (see, for example, Edelman 1993). I would suggest that both response

and intervention are associated with an interactive stance and it is in that sense that I use the terms here.

11 For details see Kramer 1994: 127–39, and Crimp and Rolston 1990.

12 Aronowitz (1995) points out that one of the crucial features by which ACT UP's history may be distinguished from previous health movements is that 'it is a movement *of* and by the victims, not merely *for* them' (377).

13 This is evident in the effectiveness (or otherwise) of various health campaigns, for instance, discussed in Chapter 3.

14 See Katharine Park (1993) for details of the case and how it was presented in the media.

15 In a recent article, Howard (1999) has argued, 'Don't throw away the condoms yet!'

16 But see Watney (1997) for a critique of the use of statistics by public health organizations and for publicity purposes.

17 This definition of ACT UP also appears on its website.

18 See also Meyer 1995.

19 See Crimp and Rolston (1990: 130–41) for full details.

20 In *Mary Kelly* (1997) Crimp makes the interesting comment that 'After I published the AIDS issue of *October* in 1997, I was accused of privileging AIDS activist art over any other aesthetic response to the epidemic. The assumption was that I was claiming that only work directly connected to movement politics had any real political force or meaning and was therefore the only work that should be supported. In fact, at that time, my argument was, rather, that activist work, agit prop, was being overlooked by art world institutions because they tenaciously held on to idealist notions of the work of art. This forced me to clarify my position, to demonstrate my commitments to other work on AIDS and to argue for other work also to be understood in political terms' (Iversen, Crimp and Bhabha 1997: 30).

21 Roland Barthes's (1977) analysis in *Image Music Text* of photography and advertising, and its connotative and denotive dimensions, remains pertinent here, despite the now slightly dated 'feel' of his position especially in relation to the idea of denotation.

22 Crimp and Rolston reference the working methods of artists Hans Haacke and Jenny Holzer as sources for the installation *Let the Record Show* (November 1987, New York Museum of Contemporary Art), underlining the instrumentalist view of art derived from a focus on political purpose which informs ACT UP's interventions: 'stealing the procedures of other artists is part of the plan – if it works, we use it' (1990: 15). In this they follow a Brechtian model of intervention which legitimates the use of other artists' work and ideas if these generate political effects and change.

23 See Haeberle (1989) for further details on that history. Significantly, *Hidden from History: Reclaiming the Gay and Lesbian Past*, the book in which this chapter appears, is dedicated 'To all those we have lost to AIDS, / and to all those struggling against it'.

24 For a full discussion of the logo see Crimp and Rolston 1990: 14–15, 17, 35. See also Meyer 1995: 59–63.

25 Saalfield and Navarro (1991) discuss this in terms of the creation of a *counter-memory*. They also discuss the issue of the appropriateness of making comparisons between the AIDS/HIV epidemic and the Holocaust.

26 One of the effects of seeing the ACT UP campaigns documented in *AIDSdemographics* is to recognize the extent to which these bodies reflect the hegemony of a certain kind of masculinity, of an older, white, middle-class male.

27 *Stonewall 25: The Making of the Lesbian and Gay Community in Britain* (1994), edited by Emma Healey and Angela Mason, provides an account of parallel experiences in the UK.

28 Such direct targeting continues to this day. See ACT UP's website <http://www.actupny.org> for details of recent actions of this kind.

29 See, for instance, Crimp and Rolston (1990: 58-9, 74, 76, 91, 94).

30 This is the case both literally (i.e. marching in the sites of power such as Wall Street) and metaphorically, through the construction of counter-discourses to challenge the eloquent silences of the Reagan government and so on.

31 Another version of this view can be found in Lorde (1984).

32 See Kimmelman (1989), for example.

33 Watney (1997) made similar points.

3

The *words* to say it[1]: HIV/AIDS in health promotion campaigns and in art

> Whoever is committed to questioning the representational determinants of AIDS ..., will have to go on to ask ... to what extent that demystificatory gesture itself, however progressively conceived, plays unwittingly into the same public spectacle that it sets out to critique. (Selden 1993: 221)

The beginnings of AIDS activist interventions among the gay and lesbian communities in the USA and the UK, as indexed by the sequencing of the chapters in this volume, predated public health promotion campaigns regarding AIDS prevention by about five to six years (Scott 1997; Watney 1997). They also predated representations of HIV/AIDS through art products, which had their heyday in the late 1980s and early 1990s, in the phase of AIDS's history when both the sense of an epidemic that might grip more than the gay community and the absence of a cure were at their strongest in western societies. In this chapter I shall discuss the representational strategies employed by predominantly UK health promotion campaigns and by artists in their attempts to visibilize HIV/AIDS, and the issue of the audiences addressed by these. I focus on health promotion campaigns and work by artists for two reasons: first, these are arenas in which cultural responses to AIDS gained prominence in the late 1980s and early 1990s; and, second, both utilize the visual field. As I shall discuss below, they do so in somewhat different ways, partly because they work to different agendas and in different sites,[2] and partly because they address audiences differently. Whereas health promotion campaigns are intended to bring about – often quite specific – change, this is not necessarily so for art work. This difference impacts on the representational strategies deployed in health promotion campaigns and in art work. A key element in these is the use of text in the visual field. The images from the health promotion campaigns and art exhibitions discussed below work to a spectrum of representation which encompasses

- text *as* image
- image *and* text
- image *without* text.[3]

Since health promotion campaigns project specific messages, they rarely present images without text. In the arts, however, the use of a *verbalized* message is more contentious and, as I shall detail below, it led to quite bitter debates about the utility and efficacy of activist art compared to other art.

A degree of contention also manifested itself in relation to the question of who should be addressed by the health campaigns and by art works, and to what purpose. Where activist art, coming from within the gay community, often addressed either public institutions or the gay community itself with specific messages, other art work had a less clearly defined audience or message and could thus create the impression of a diffusion or absence of political will. The health promotion campaigns aimed at reducing risk of HIV infection among the general population and produced campaigns for a range of audiences. The agendas informing these campaigns at the level of the image and the audience were, as I shall indicate, very different from those of the activists in the gay community. Health promotion campaigns and art works produced in response to HIV/AIDS were all concerned with visibilizing HIV/AIDS but they did so in diverse and (sometimes internally) contradictory ways, signalling a general uncertainty regarding the most effective way to intervene.

Mainstreaming AIDS: health promotion campaigns in the late 1980s and early 1990s

When the health promotion campaigns in the UK began in 1986 (Field, Wellings and McVey 1997: 6) they utilized a representational strategy familiar from work such as ACT UP's, namely the conjoining of the verbal and the visual to propagate a particular message. The use of 'words' is integral to health promotion campaigns which, after all, are designed to project a particular message. The messages spelt out in the AIDS prevention campaigns, however, were significantly different from those produced by ACT UP and other AIDS activist groups. I shall begin by analysing this difference which is, of course, partly a function of the messages coming precisely from those institutions which had been the objects of attack by gay AIDS activists for their inactivity in responding to the AIDS crisis.

AIDS prevention work by public health organizations was fuelled by agendas aligned with mainstream politics rather than by the agendas of the gay community such as 'drugs into bodies' (see previous chapter). It was concerned with the notion that 'in order to be credible and effective the campaigns [had to] be seen by their target audience to be relevant and motivating, *whilst not causing offence to the wider population*' (Field, Wellings and McVey 1997: 11; emphasis added). 'Offence to the wider population' is notoriously difficult to define since it is often specific, vociferous groups, particular news media and tabloids such as the *Sun* or individuals like Mary Whitehouse in the UK (Watney 1994: 129), or the Christian moral right in the USA, who become the 'voice' of some imaginary 'wider population'. However, mainstream and thus of necessity heterosexual concerns, particularly in the conservative climate of the 1980s (Smith 1994), underpinned the work of the HEA (Health Education Authority) in the UK from the beginning.[4] Significantly, and predictably, their campaigns surfaced at a point when the fact that AIDS was not just 'a gay plague' became established. As Peter Scott (1997) maintains: 'from 1986/87 governments began to be concerned about the possibility of a heterosexual epidemic. They threw money at the problem and a vast new HIV prevention industry grew up almost overnight' (305). Watney (1997) has pointed out that 'uncertainty about the future course of heterosexual transmission was entirely understandable in the 1980s' (84) but this does not in and of itself account for the specificities of the AIDS prevention campaigns of the UK HEA during that phase.

Imaging AIDS in health promotion campaigns

In visibilizing AIDS, the initial tactic of the HEA was to address the general population in mass media campaigns which were intended to raise awareness about HIV/AIDS. This awareness-raising often did not go beyond the point of naming AIDS, thus reinforcing the ignorance of the 'general population' it was seeking to address. It was not aimed at identifying either particular groups of people or specific practices with HIV/AIDS. The first public AIDS awareness campaign 'used television and posters featuring icebergs and tombstones' (Field, Wellings and McVey 1997: 6). It thus depersonalized HIV/AIDS, divorcing it from bodies and from sex. In the subsequent campaign, 'AIDS: Don't Die of Ignorance', the precedent was set for using text *as* image, a strategy which continued the depersonalization of HIV/AIDS and which the

HEA employed throughout the late 1980s and early 1990s. Text thus became the means to message for several HEA campaigns. The advantage of this strategy was to move away from the stigmatizing identification of specific people with HIV/AIDS. The disadvantage was that it enabled viewers to dissociate themselves from the message since it offered no image of themselves as being specifically implicated in the HIV/AIDS epidemic. King (1990) maintains that part of the ineffectualness of the HEA anti-AIDS campaigns was this dissociation of HIV/AIDS from people: 'The role of media campaigns should be to support peer education efforts within affected communities. State educational programmes originate, by definition, outside of any community.'

The demand of the HEA's 1987 campaign, 'AIDS: Don't Die of Ignorance', disregarded the fact that knowledge about AIDS was a relative matter.[5] Whilst many gay men and gay activists in particular had developed substantial levels of knowledge about HIV/AIDS, general levels of ignorance about AIDS,[6] not just in the population at large but among, for instance, health workers[7] as well, were extensive.[8] The HEA's initial consciousness-raising exercise, which suggested that ignorance equals death and, by implication, knowledge equals life, presented a view of AIDS unsupported by what knowledge there was about HIV/AIDS at the time. It did not, for instance, take into account what was known about who might be at risk. However, it very clearly aligned AIDS with death. The specificity of the message, though juxtaposed with the reality of the indeterminacy of the disease, recreated the notion of the government and the HEA *as authority*,[9] speaking to anonymous, depersonalized others[10] who had everyman status by virtue of their non-specificity.[11] The potential for dissociation and the othering of HIV/AIDS (AIDS is what happens to others and is other from me) was thus immense.

'You're as safe as you want to be': voluntarism, individualism, choice and risk in HEA campaigns

From December 1988 to September 1989, the HEA ran their 'You're as safe as you want to be' campaigns.[12] Two types of images were used: text as image and images of people combined with text. Where text was the image (e.g. Figure 5) the strategy of featuring white script on a black background, familiar from the 'AIDS: Don't Die of Ignorance' campaign, was continued. This presented an eye-catching picture based upon contrast and the notion of issues being black-and-white. It belied, however, the reality of HIV/AIDS, the state of knowledge about it, and the reality of who was (being) infected (Watney 1994: 48–61). The

WHAT IS THE DIFFERENCE BETWEEN HIV AND AIDS?

TIME.

HIV (Human Immunodeficiency Virus) is the virus which leads to AIDS.

It is now recognised that most people who are infected with this virus will go on to develop AIDS.

It may take 1 year. It may take 5 years. It may take 15 years.

During this time a person can look and feel perfectly healthy.

But, through sexual intercourse, they could pass on the virus to others.

It is estimated that for every person with AIDS there are thirty with HIV.

Obviously, the more people you sleep with the more likely you are to become infected.

But the answer doesn't just mean fewer sexual partners.

It also means using a condom, or even having sex that avoids penetration.

AIDS may be incurable but it's also avoidable.

AIDS. YOU'RE AS SAFE AS YOU WANT TO BE.

FOR MORE INFORMATION OR CONFIDENTIAL ADVICE ABOUT AIDS FREEPHONE THE 24 HOUR NATIONAL AIDS HELPLINE ON 0800 567123

5 *What is the difference between HIV and AIDS? Time.*
(December 1988–September 1989)

issues were not as black and white or as clear cut as these images suggested. But the simple, instantly absorbable message was, for example, 'What is the difference between HIV and AIDS? Time.'[13] That message, presented as a white-on-black block occupying most of the page, was supported by a black-on-white base in which further commentary on the statement presented in the central block was offered. This declared that 'It is now recognised that *most* people who are infected with this virus will go on to develop AIDS. It *may* take 1 year. It *may* take 5 years. It *may* take 15 years. During this time a person *can* look and feel perfectly healthy. But, through sexual intercourse, they *could* pass on the virus to others. It is *estimated* ...' (emphasis added). As shown above, the inevitability of the sequence – HIV leads to AIDS in time – was qualified in the additional supporting text on the posters, supplied in much smaller typeface than the central message. However, it did require the reading of that second block to understand the relativity of the white-on-black statement that appeared so authoritative.[14]

Authoritative assertion was also the tone used in this campaign in the appeal to individual responsibility which was again writ larger than the explaining black-on-white section: 'AIDS: You're as safe as you want to be'. The certainty with which the notion 'you are as safe as you want to be' was expressed – underwritten by the use of the indicative and the present tense – introduced a voluntaristic (as safe as you *want* to be) and thus an individualized (it's up to *you*) element into the issue of the acquisition of HIV/AIDS as well as the notion of choice and also of risk (being at risk as an implicit matter of choice).[15] All four, voluntarism, individualism, choice and risk, were mainstays of the conservative politics of the 1980s.[16] In appealing to these notions, the campaign promoted an ideology which privatized individuals' relation to AIDS, making AIDS a matter of their personal choice.

'You're as safe as you want to be' projected the idea that you could be and were responsible for what happened to you.[17] This message was reinforced by the HEA's February to September 1988 campaign, with the slogan, 'AIDS -You Know the Risks, the Decision is Yours'. The campaign, run on television and posters, featured a young woman and a young man about to make the decision to have sex or spend the night together. It was thus heterosexually invested, aiming at 'young people who are sexually active and outside a long-term or monogamous relationship' (Field, Wellings and McVey 1997: 14). One version focused on the man as the decision-maker,[18] the other on the woman.[19]

My Place Screen: There is still no cure for AIDS and it's on the increase; you can't tell by looking who's infected. *Man: 'Do you want to go and sit down?'. Screen*: The more partners you have, the greater the risk; using a condom could help save your life. *Man: 'Do you fancy coming back to my place?'. Screen:* AIDS. You know the risks, the decision is yours.

Stay Screen: There is still no cure for AIDS and it's on the increase; both men and women can pass on the virus through sex. *Woman: 'Would you like some coffee?'. Screen:* You can't tell by looking who's infected; the more partners you have, the greater the risk; using a condom could help save your life. *Woman: 'It's quite late. Will you stay?'. Screen:* AIDS. You know the risks, the decision is yours. (Field, Wellings and McVey 1997: 14)[20]

These two different versions of the same campaign produced subtly different representations of women and men and their relation to heterosex, with different, gendered types of normative behaviour. The encounter in the first version which featured the man as the one making the advance and the woman as respondent – and therefore, here, as the person to make the decision – was set in a public context, *his* place being equated with sex. In the second section the two were already in *her* place, a private context in which he was placed into the position of making the decision. The assumption seemed to be that going to a man's place equalled having sex and staying at a woman's place (rather than going to her place) equalled sex. In the March 1988 to December 1989 campaign the woman was always presented as the passive recipient of the man's sexual attention.[21] This was clearly not regarded as conflicting with the notion that the woman might be (pro)active and have a choice in whether or not to have sex and in whether or not to use condoms as suggested in the 1988 campaign cited above. Yet the evidence regarding actual heterosexual practice is that many women do not feel able to make choices about what happens in a heterosexual encounter (Holland *et al.* 1992, 1994a).

Much more might be said on the particular and gendered nature of these campaigns. The issue I want to focus on here, however, is the assumption that having sex and everything that goes with it is a private, unarticulated decision[22] made by the individual on her or his own. This assumption reinforces the notion of sex as taboo, i.e. as unspoken,[23] and as an individual matter of choice, placing the decision to expose yourself to AIDS ('You know the risks, the decision is yours') on the individual woman or man, and making that person implicitly responsible for having AIDS, should she or he catch it.

In later campaigns this line was altered. Images of heterosexual couples in intimate embrace carried underneath them the slogan, 'And they don't know each other well enough to discuss using a condom?' (Field, Wellings, McVey 1997: 16). This suggested that the use of the condom was a matter of explicit negotiation between people as opposed to a matter of unarticulated, private resolution. The presumably supposedly rhetorical question, 'And they don't know each other well enough to discuss using a condom?', ostensibly sought to promote discussions between sexually active heterosexual couples about condom use. But its deriding stance failed to acknowledge both the persistence in mainstream cultural representation of sex as an activity which is beyond articulacy[24] or articulation,[25] and the issue of power differentials between young women and men in their sexual encounters with each other.[26]

Three campaigns under the banner 'You're as safe as you want to be' were run specifically for young people, a group targeted in general advertising, especially of the 1980s and early 1990s, as risk-takers. Specifically in the arena of advertising for smoking,[27] but not only there, risk-taking as a desirable thing to do, proving one's resistance, resilience, self-reliance and sheer dare-devil mentality, was one of the key features of western culture in the 1980s and early 1990s. Risk was used in those ads, not as a deterrent but as an incitement to transcend certain boundaries. By utilizing the statement 'You're as safe as you want to be' the HEA campaigns of 1988–89 were addressing a youth audience through playing off recognizable tropes from youth advertising but effectively sending out the opposite message from what, one imagines, was intended.[28] Additionally, they failed to recognize that notions of risk and safety carry very different meanings for women and men.

The continued displacement of responsibility for HIV infection ('You're as safe as you want to be') on to the heterosexual individual addressed in these campaigns is, of course, the mirror image of the notion of 'bringing it on yourself' which had been levelled at the gay community (see Watney 1997: 83–6). It suggested that those who suffered from AIDS were directly responsible for their condition, that they had not wanted to be safe and had deliberately exposed themselves to the disease. As such it contributed to the blame culture which accompanied reactions to the discovery of the AIDS epidemic.[29] Blame and fear were two key elements in the early AIDS campaigns by the UK HEA: fear as a source of generating avoidance behaviour; blame as a means of attributing responsibility. In the process AIDS functioned as the third term, the other which in and of itself was not visible but waited on the other side of what you could not see. A number of anti-AIDS campaigns were run using precisely that notion of AIDS as the third, invisible term. Best known of these is perhaps the December 1988 to March 1989 campaign featuring two identical black-and-white images of a beautiful woman on two separate, successive pages of various magazines. The first image had the caption, 'If this woman had the virus which leads to AIDS, in a few years she could look like the person over the page'. The second, identical image was captioned 'Worrying isn't it'. Further text underneath this image pointed out that 'A person can be infected with HIV for several years before it shows any signs or symptoms'. The relegation of the person to the dehumanized 'it' (since 'it' is ambiguously deployed here as a possible referent for both 'a person' and 'HIV') is an amazing slip/(page) in a presentation which, in time-honoured fashion, constructs woman as the carrier of deadly diseases and as the other whose appearance belies her 'true' nature.[30] This inability to see due to the lack of a distinguishing mark in those who are HIV-positive is here constructed as having the effect of placing AIDS in our midst, socializing it into the position of the 'enemy within', the 'hidden enemy' of the spy stories of the Cold War[31] which function as one element in the citational cultural chain on which this imaging relies. The suspicion of others evoked in this representation points to a sociophobia, already indexed by the silent, individual decision-making which figured in the earlier campaigns, which is both anti-social and anti-sexual in its implications. Since, as these campaigns suggest, you cannot trust anyone, everybody is a potential carrier[32] and you are at risk, your only form of reliance is self-reliance. The obvious problem with this kind of campaign is that it on the one hand constructs AIDS as a disease acquired in an emotionally and sexually charged *social* context but, on the other, sets up that context as one which is not negotiated between or among individuals but in which people act individually rather than in a socially interrelating manner.

Confusing categories: bodies at risk

However, the focus on *people* was one way in which the 'You're as safe as you want to be' campaigns were different from the previous ones. While the verbally encoded message projected a specific line about AIDS prevention, the focus on couples offered new points of identification in the form of the depiction of specific individuals to the target (and, indeed, other) audiences. The people depicted (Figure 6) were invariably young, beautiful, white, heterosexual, seemingly economically secure, sexually active, assumed to perceive themselves as agents capable of changing their situation and behaviour,[33] presumably healthy but in need of protecting themselves. These early campaigns by the HEA were thus directed at a very particular group of people whom these campaigns were seeking to preserve. In contrast to, for instance, ACT UP's activism which significantly focused on those living with AIDS and their needs, prominently demanding that public bodies should take responsibility for their care, these campaigns concentrated on those presumed not to have AIDS (yet) and worked on risk-elimination through focusing on individual responsibility. The person with AIDS, already iconically established as the dying, homosexual, emaciated individual,[34] was now juxtaposed with the healthy, 'at risk' body, object of a non-specific, invisible yet omnipresent threat.

Gilman (1988b) highlights the absence of the diseased body in the representation of AIDS in health campaigns (106) and the concomitant focus on the healthy and frequently beautiful body as the 'at risk' body in need of protection. This focus has to be understood within a context where the HEA were seeking to countermand the use in the popular media and tabloid press of images of people suffering from advanced stages of AIDS-related illnesses. Gilman argues that this focus led to the stigmatization of the HIV-positive body which cannot be shown, or can be shown only as a site of suffering. Visualization and visibility in the general cultural field, within mainstream, non-specialized (i.e. non-medicalized) contexts, answer to those conventions and idealizations of the representation of the body which conjoin the aesthetic with the moral, separating those who are 'sick' from those who are 'healthy'.[35] Only the latter may be represented, and only the latter, the HEA campaigns suggest, deserve protection. The campaigns were thus not working for those already infected but targeted assumed at-risk groups, projecting the notion that those addressed by the campaigns were not yet infected.

Two examples demonstrate the impact of this kind of campaigning. The first relates to a story told by Michael Bronski (1997) about a 'safer sex crisis' experienced by an AIDS educator who, when cottaging, found that 'As he was about to make his move and go down on the man – things have to happen quickly in a public bathroom patrolled by the police – he saw that the man's face was covered with KS lesions' (126). Despite believing that 'sucking cock without ejaculation is a safe activity' the man hesitated to proceed. 'Why should he hesitate to go down on someone with visible KS when he has probably, unknowingly, gone down on men with similar conditions?' (126). Bronski uses this story as one example of the problematic impact undifferentiated health promotion campaigns for gay men have on homosexuals many of whom, as Bronski's evidence shows, still have unsafe sex. The fetishization of the beautiful body in HEA AIDS prevention campaigns, including the beautiful male body in campaigns targeted at gay men (Figure 7), sends problematic messages to a community already in many respects overly imbued with a focus on the body as asset.[36] Bronski argues that this is because these campaigns raise issues of identification and desire by conflating beauty and health on the one hand, and lack

HOW FAR WILL YOU GO BEFORE YOU MENTION CONDOMS?

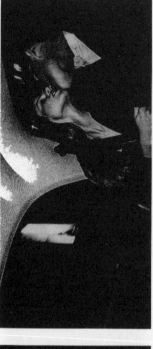

THIS FAR?

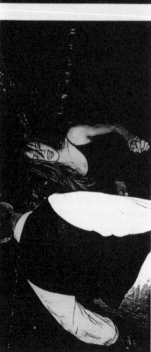

THIS FAR?

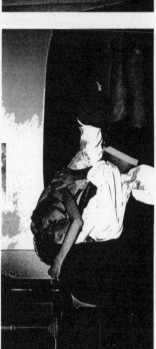

THIS FAR?

THIS FAR?

Today, no one can ignore the need to mention condoms. Have sex with someone without using one and not only could you risk an unwanted pregnancy, but you also risk contracting one of the many sexually transmitted diseases.

Like Herpes, Chlamydia, Gonorrhoea, and of course HIV, the virus which leads to AIDS.

So the question isn't if, but when you mention condoms. You could mention them at any moment leading up to sexual intercourse. In reality, it's not quite so easy.

Mention them too early and you might feel you look pushy or unavailable. Leave it too late and you risk getting so carried away you might not mention them at all.

Where is the easiest moment to say you want to use one? How about while you're still wearing your knickers? In this instance it would be perfect the picture there.

By now you've gone far enough to make it obvious that you both want to have sex. But not so far that you're in danger of getting emotionally and sexually carried away.

It's a perfect opportunity. So take it. Say you want to use a condom.

Say he hasn't got one? Well have one of your own at the ready just in case. It really doesn't matter whose you use.

And then you can go just as far as you like.

FOR MORE INFORMATION OR ADVICE ABOUT AIDS OR HIV, PHONE THE FREE NATIONAL AIDS HELPLINE ON 0800 567 123. IT'S OPEN 24 HOURS A DAY AND IS COMPLETELY CONFIDENTIAL.

of beauty and ill-health on the other. The campaigns simultaneously and contradictorily suggest that those depicted – with whom the viewer is presumably invited to identify – are healthy, if at risk, while unseen others are ill. If those depicted are not ill, however, why should they use a condom with each other? 'Thus there emerges a cognitive dissonance between the popular designation of positive men as "deadly" and health promotion's representation of them as potential partners in "hot, safe, sex"' (Bronski 1997: 123). The difficulty of deciding what to avoid and what not to avoid undermines effective decision-making[37] in sexual encounters. This is made worse by the failure of health promotion campaigns to address HIV-negative and HIV-positive people in ways which acknowledge the differences in their status.[38] Both Bronski and Odets (1997) suggest that simply advocating condom use for all is inadequate. Odets argues that by reducing 'prevention to a set of concrete, universal instructions that never [speak] (that cannot speak) of motivation, purposes, or outcome' (136), the AIDS prevention campaigns fail to address their target audiences, both those who are not infected and those who are infected. In consequence there is little incentive to follow AIDS prevention measures. Odets (1997) states that 'Among psychotherapy patients who decide to test after long periods of indecision, I have fairly consistently seen behavioural changes in only a single group. These are men who believed, felt, or feared they were HIV-positive and then actually tested negative. These men often dramatically lower their potential exposure to HIV because they suddenly feel that they do, after all, have something to protect' (138).

The second example, indicating the negative impact of the privileging of certain kinds of bodies in mainstream culture, relates to the case in the UK in 1997 of a prize-winning photo by Richard Sawdon Smith of a man dying from AIDS (Figure 8). The photo which won the Kobal Portrait Prize showed the man nude, standing with his head bowed and holding on to a walking stick. His downward gaze directed the viewer's eyes towards his enlarged scrotum and slightly deformed legs. The contrast between the man's nude body and the dark, undifferentiated background, as well as the fact that his genitals occupied the centre of the photo, reinforced the focus on his body and in particular, his enlarged scrotum. *The Times*, the newspaper which sponsored the exhibition in London's National Portrait Gallery where the photo was shown, decided not to publish the picture in the paper since it was judged to be 'too disturbing'. This prompted *The Guardian* to publish the photo as the 'Picture of the week' (27 September 1997),

facing] **6** *How far will you go ...?* (July 1992–March 1993)

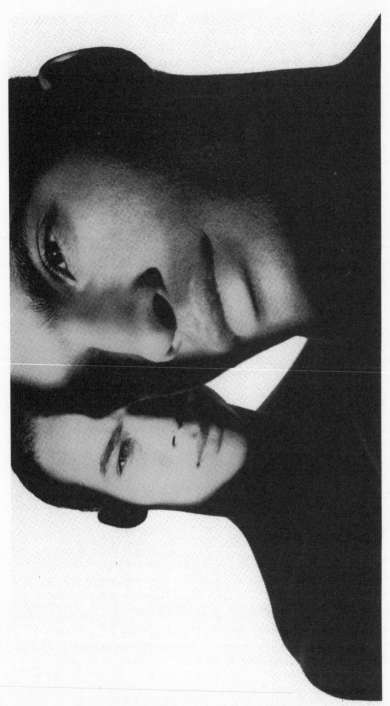

THEY DON'T HAVE SAFER SEX JUST BECAUSE IT'S SAFER.

Sex.

We all know how much we enjoy it.

So why should our attitudes change when it comes to safer sex? After all, people were enjoying it long before the

By safer sex we simply mean any activity where infected blood or semen (or vaginal fluid) can't enter your body.

Mutual masturbation, fingering, massage or body rubbing

But there are plenty of others you won't have, and half the fun is finding new ways to enjoy each other.

Anal sex, however, is still the highest risk activity and even using a condom won't make it completely safe.

safer sex leaflet (available from gay bars and clubs), or ring your local helpline.

Alternatively call the National AIDS Helpline free of charge on 0800 567 123. It's open 24 hours complete with commentary. According to that commentary, the National Portrait Gallery's director, Charles Saumarez Smith, who was among the judges, said that the photo stood out as 'classically austere'.[39] He also said that 'when the image was selected none of the judges knew that it depicted a medical condition associated with AIDS.' ('Picture of the week': 2). It is unclear what the status of this comment is, whether it is meant to 'excuse' the choice or to justify it. The photographer, Richard Sawdon Smith,[40] meanwhile raised questions about *The Times*'s use of the word 'disturbing', pointing out that 'They've printed pictures of starving children in Africa or bloody corpses from war-torn parts of Europe. How could a sympathetic portrait of a sick man be more disturbing than those?' ('Picture of the week': 2). The obvious answer, when comparing the portrait with the AIDS prevention campaign images produced by the HEA is, of course, that the realistic portrayal of a full frontal nude male focusing on the enlarged scrotum is not permissible in a culture where firstly only the beautiful, that is healthy, body may be presented within mainstream cultural sites (as opposed to selected audiences), and where, moreover, the portrayal of male genitals is the object of censorship.[41]

A question of audience: differences in health promotion campaigns for gays, straights and others

The problematic of how to image male sexuality also presented itself in the campaigns the HEA ran for gay and bisexual men, most of which were disseminated through the gay press and so-called male-interest magazines. As I shall discuss below, this problematic was addressed by creating pictures which, in many respects, borrowed their representational styles from images circulating in cultural products aimed at heterosexuals. Much critique has been levelled at mainstream organizations both for waiting to intervene in the AIDS crisis until it was deemed to have become a heterosexual concern, and then for directing almost all interventionist energies towards heterosexuals rather than homosexuals or bisexual men, to date and throughout the crisis the group in western culture with the highest rate of new HIV infections and AIDS (Scott 1997; Watney 1997). When the HEA did begin to run campaigns for gay and bisexual men from December 1988, it did so for the most part by circulating campaigns in media aimed at a specifically gay and possibly bisexual readership. This tactic was something of a double-edged sword since on the one hand it reinforced

facing] **7** *They don't …* (October 1989–March 1990)

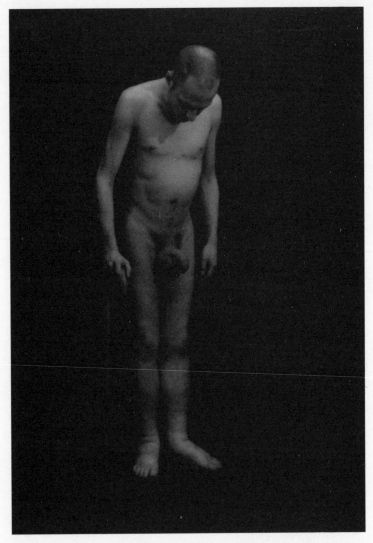

8 *Portrait of Simon* (1997)

the them-and-us mentality which had been so destructive in the early stages of the emergence of AIDS through its construction of gay men (as opposed to heterosexuals) as carriers and victims of the 'gay plague', but, on the other hand, it tried to reach its intended target groups by addressing them specifically through the media those groups were thought to access in particular. The campaigns aimed at gay men as much as those addressing heterosexuals, however, reinforced the cultural boundaries between homosexual and heterosexual territories,

aligning mainstream television and the national press with heterosexuals, and the gay press and male-interest magazines with homosexuals,
perpetuating the invisibilization of homosexuals in dominant cultural
representation. Discussing the relationship of the development of circulation of information in contemporary western society and the atom-
ization of that society through the fragmentation of groups, individuals
and traditions, Michel de Certeau (1997) argues that 'to inform means,
first of all, to overcome the resistances of a place and the opacities that
belong to it for the sake of producing a system of transparence' (91).
The HEA campaigns both challenged *and* reinforced those resistances
(e.g. the use of condoms) selectively through maintaining notions of
specific cultural sites for people with different sexual orientations and
through the use of particular citational chains such as hetero-romance
and other forms of popular culture to present particular views of who
was at risk from HIV/AIDS, who needed protecting from it and how.

People from diverse ethnic backgrounds were ignored by the HEA
campaigns until 1992 when a national AIDS awareness campaign for
people from eight different cultural and linguistic groups was
launched. The campaign utilized the radio and the local and minority
ethnic press. The press campaign combined image with extensive text.
Entitled 'Facts You Need to Know – HIV and AIDS', the campaign
sought to provide information about HIV/AIDS both 'in English and
also in the relevant language for Bengali, Gujarati, Hindi, Punjabi,
Urdu, Cantonese, Swahili, Arabic (and African/Caribbean) groups'
(Field, Wellings and McVey 1997: 25). One image presented a healthy,
happy smiling Indian family; another a young Indian couple. In these
images the women tended to wear traditional dress, e.g. saris, while the
men were dressed in western clothes. Some work might be done on the
implications of the cultural construction of these groupings for the
effectiveness of the campaigns. As with the campaigns aimed at white
audiences, however, the bodies presented were the seemingly healthy,
as yet uninfected bodies which implicitly needed protection.

Field, Wellings and McVey (1997: 39–40) record some interesting
findings from the evaluation of this campaign, which was discontinued
very quickly. These include the fact that awareness and knowledge
about HIV and AIDS was high among the sample group of Caribbean
origin because of 'a "sensitivity" to the commonly made media connection between Africa and AIDS' (39) and owing to English being the
first language for many from this group. This meant that they had
already gleaned information about HIV/AIDS from other mainstream
media. A further finding from the evaluation of this campaign was that
'Arabic groups ... demonstrated a sensitivity to individual targeting'

(39). In fact, not only Arabs, but people from other ethnic minorities did not like being singled out in these campaigns. Not surprisingly, they experienced this as stigmatizing. Field, Wellings and McVey also note 'significant differences in access to and willingness to take on board HIV and AIDS messages' (1997: 40). This is in part accounted for through resistance to the implicit stigmatizing discussed above and its refusal by the targeted groups, but also by high levels of illiteracy among certain groups and particularly women, and women's more restricted access to various media. A campaign which relies on text to convey its message will not reach those who cannot read, and if the image provides no clue as to the message – as was the case with this campaign – little is achieved. Most importantly, though, 'the research findings led to uncertainty as to whether mass media campaigns specifically targeted at these communities would remain the most effective way to reach black and minority ethnic groups'[42] since 'singling out certain groups on ethnic grounds using mass media may be counter productive and perhaps stigmatizing' (Field, Wellings and McVey 1997: 40). The consequence of this perception was that from 1992 'black and minority ethnic groups [were] targeted through community level initiatives and leaflets and other materials … made available in community languages' (Field, Wellings and McVey 1997: 40).

This cultural separatism, with its concomitant benefits and limitations was reinforced by later campaigns, specifically in the arena of groups with diverse sexual orientations. As Field, Wellings and McVey (1997) put it: 'The campaign targeting gay and bisexual men … continued to run through the gay press, listings and male interest titles and [covered] issues in a way that would not be relevant to a wider audience' (8). Quite what is meant by covering issues 'in a way that would not be relevant to a wider audience' remains unclear. But the campaigns on safer sex aimed at condom use[43] reveal the discrepancies perceived to exist between heterosexual and homosexual sexual behaviour. In these campaigns differences in sexual behaviour are, on the one hand, assumed to transcend the stigmatizing of specific *groups of people* as opposed to particular behaviour and sexual practices as sources of HIV infection or transmission. On the other, assumptions are made about sexual practices in different groups of people that may well ignore the realities of sexual encounters in such groups (see Wilton 1994: 86). The HEA campaigns about condom use for gay men, for example, used images such as a condom being pulled lengthwise by two hands, or two hands opening the wrapper of a condom, or a condom lying on a shelf above a radiator by a switched-on lamp, which could, in fact, have appeared in any heterosexually oriented mainstream magazine or newspaper. The differentiating moment was thus not the image or indeed the headline message, which was 'Is yours up to it?', 'Rip off the wrapper. Open with care', and 'Sometimes things can get too hot for a condom' respectively, but the vocabulary used in the accompanying text which provided further information about condom use, utilizing words and phrases which, one assumes, were regarded as inappropriate in a heterosexual context since they never appeared in the parallel condom-based campaigns aimed at heterosexuals. The phrases in question were 'So if you're going to fuck ...' and 'A bit of rough handling may not matter to jeans' (Figures 9 and 10). These references to sexual intercourse and practices in colloquial language had no equivalent in the campaigns for heterosexuals. Campaigns which addressed sexual practices were directed at gay men as if only gay men used a diversity of sexual practices, or indeed any, in their sexual encounters. The white-on-black 1993 campaign (Figure 11) which stated 'Oral sex. Raunchy. But risky?', for instance, aimed only at gay men. After stating that 'anal sex without a condom is far more risky', the text supporting the white-on-black block explained, 'certain things may increase the risk from oral sex. If he comes in your mouth, for instance. Particularly if you have cuts or sores in your mouth, bleeding gums or gingivitis. There's also a possibility that HIV can be passed on in pre-cum.' Such explicitness did not materialize in the campaigns aimed at heterosexuals. Tellingly, sexual practice was never raised as an issue in campaigns aimed at heterosexuals, where the missionary position and vaginal penetration appeared to be the non-spoken norm.[44] Here the sanitizing of sex deflected from actual practice to decorous inarticulacy which, in consequence, simultaneously normalized such non-specificity and invisibilized the actuality of heterosexual sexual practices.

The condom-centred campaigns aimed at gay men contained specific information, again at the verbal rather than the image level, about lubricants and the detrimental impact of oil and heat on condoms, neither of which was regarded as an issue in heterosexual contexts.[45] Yet it is clearly the case that massage oils, lubricants and heat from lamps, radiators etc. are used and have the same effects on condoms whether in a homosexual or in a heterosexual sexual encounter. At the level of the word rather than the image, then, the campaigns aimed at gay and bisexual men were more explicit about the specificities of condom use in sexual contexts than they were in campaigns for heterosexuals.[46] In the latter the main focus was on when the issue of condom use should be raised in a romantic encounter which leads to sex and by whom rather than on the 'appropriate' handling of condoms. The assumption that gay men need educating in the treatment of condoms in ways that heterosexuals do not is erroneous, and ignores the needs of both groups for full information about this issue. It also reinforces and constructs views of the sexual behaviour and relations of gays and heterosexuals which do not necessarily coincide with the realities of those experiences (Wellings *et al.* 1994). As Miller (1993), for example, points out: 'sodomy ... is probably the least specific practice in the whole history of sexuality' (214). Where the condom-centred campaigns run by the HEA for homosexuals focused on the condom and in many instances did not use people as part of the image, most campaigns related to condom use aimed at heterosexuals pictured individuals and specific sexual occasions. Condom use was thus socialized in the heterosexual context (see Figure 12) while it remained functionalized within the homosexual one. The underlying assumption was that where the social outweighed the functional in a heterosexual sexual encounter, the same was not true for a homosexual one.

This sent out messages which contradicted other campaigns, directed at gays and run contemporaneously, that utilized images of men but drew heavily on heterosexual romantic iconography. Thus one

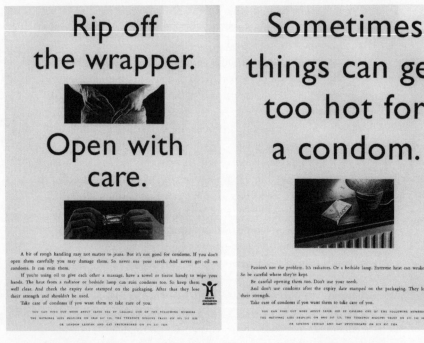

9, 10 *Rip off the wrapper* (August 1992–November 1993), *Sometimes ...*
(August 1992–March 1993)

image which was used repeatedly in campaigns aimed at gay men between December 1988 and 1996 (Figure 13) was of two men whose naked upper torsos[47] were visible (no cocks or buttocks here). One man was placed lower than the other and thus positioned in a 'feminine' place, leaning against the background figure, in a representation of soft-focus romance and intimacy which privileges a couple relationship of the kind portrayed in some teenage magazines or on the covers of

Oral sex.
Raunchy.
But risky?

At the moment, no one can say for sure what the level of risk of HIV infection from oral sex may be.

While it's a fact that anal sex without a condom is far more risky, it's thought that certain things may increase the risk from oral sex.

If he comes in your mouth, for instance. Particularly if you have cuts or sores in your mouth, bleeding gums or gingivitis.

There's also a possibility that HIV can be passed on in pre-cum. So for added reassurance and protection, you can use a condom.

Choose one that has a kitemark on the pack. And if you aren't keen on the taste of condoms, try the mint flavoured variety.

Unfortunately there are no absolute answers about oral sex.

But if you like, you can talk it over with someone who may be able to help with any further questions.

Call either The National AIDS Helpline free on 0800 567 123, The Terrence Higgins Trust on 071 242 1010 or London Lesbian and Gay Switchboard on 071 837 7324.

11 Oral sex (1993)

AND THEY DON'T KNOW EACH OTHER WELL ENOUGH TO DISCUSS USING A CONDOM?

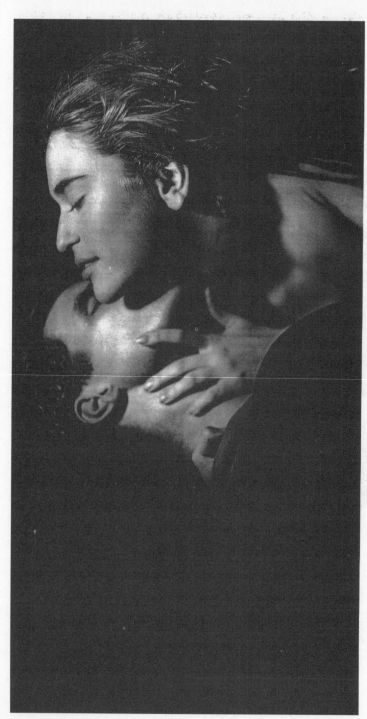

You know someone well enough to go to bed with them.

You know someone well enough to let them explore every inch of your body.

And then you don't know them well enough to discuss using a condom? Ridiculous isn't it?

But it happens. And it needn't.

A condom can help stop you getting HIV.

This is the Human Immunodeficiency Virus that leads to AIDS.

Someone can have HIV for several years without knowing it.

They can look and feel perfectly healthy, but through unprotected sex, they can pass on the virus to you.

So if you choose to have sex, make sure you use a condom. Talk about it today. And never, ever, feel embarrassed.

Because if you feel awkward now, you could feel a whole lot worse later.

AIDS YOU'RE AS SAFE AS YOU WANT TO BE

certain kinds of pulp romances where structural inequalities between heterosexual couples and an undefined yearning which evades sexual realities are the norm (Duncombe and Marsden 1995; Jackson 1995; Langford 1995). As Gilman (1997) puts it: 'the visual vocabulary employed comes from the erotic vocabulary of mass advertising ... [These images] refuse to treat sex as sex' (112).

Given the representational inadequacies of many health promotion campaigns, and since the effectiveness of these campaigns depends on their being 'seen by their target audience to be relevant and motivating' (Field, Wellings and McVey 1997: 11), it may well be the case that, as the HEA strategy on HIV and AIDS health promotion suggests, 'Community-based and self-help voluntary organisations are well placed to develop targeted health promotion work. Some of this work, safer sex intiatives for example, may be better undertaken by these groups rather than by the government or its agencies' (Field, Wellings and McVey 1997: 11). This is reinforced by the fact that peer education is generally a more effective tool for achieving change than top-down general campaigns. However, without adequate resourcing such work is not possible. Inadequate resourcing has been a serious problem for health promotion issues in the gay community. There are a number of reasons for this lack of resources. Watney (1997) points to the fact that the specific construction of narratives of epidemiological data which obscures the rise of HIV infections among gay men in favour of a different 'story' has contributed significantly to the chronic under-funding of AIDS prevention work done by community-based groups. Scott (1997) views the the de-gaying of HIV/AIDS prevention work as critical in this context. Indeed, Scott goes so far as to state that 'state-sponsored HIV prevention has done more harm than good' (305) since that prevention regime has targeted too little funding at gay men and has been led by a heterosexist agenda. But HIV/AIDS is, of course, not just a gay men's issue. Many contributors to *Acting on AIDS* (1997) understand, as the editors put it, 'AIDS in its specificity, as a series of many different epidemics, each situated at the intersection of local and global politics, culture and demographics' (Oppenheimer and Reckitt 1997: 2). Oppenheimer and Reckitt rightly point out that the previous notion of 'a single, global epidemic is profoundly unhelpful to those who are interested in implementing prevention, treatment, and care programmes designed to minimize the harm caused by AIDS to actual communities' (2). However, the understanding of HIV/AIDS as a series of different epidemics also creates its own difficulties since it atomizes

facing] **12** *And they don't know each other well enough ...?* (December 1988–November 1989)

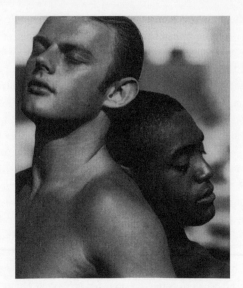

CHOOSE SAFER SEX.

FOR CONFIDENTIAL ADVICE FREEPHONE THE 24 HOUR NATIONAL AIDS HELPLINE ON 0800 567 123.

13 *Choose safer sex* (March–May 1990)

HIV/AIDS into different epidemics. This generates exactly the kind of 'liberal tolerance for the diversity of people with AIDS, a broad commitment to offering resources to fight AIDS in the poorer countries, and a diffuse resolve to get on with bringing the epidemic[s] under control' (2) which Oppenheimer and Reckitt attribute only to a position which understands AIDS as a single epidemic. In 1999, for example, HIV/AIDS was off the mainstream media agenda. There are no significant prevention campaigns which reach the 'general public' any more; HIV/AIDS is not much talked about. It is as if HIV/AIDS had ceased to affect the 'general public'. Occasional reports of new developments in the treatment of AIDS or HIV prevention are the most one ever hears. In the UK, at least, there is a strong sense that the HIV prevention campaigns 'effectively reinscribed boundaries of the various western national communities – white nuclear families [are] on the inside, while those actually effected by AIDS [are] positioned on the outside' (Oppenheimer and Reckitt 1997: 2). This is particularly worrying in a context where, as Field, Wellings and McVey suggest, 'people may, in the absence of any visible signs of the disease, use high levels of media activity as a proxy measure of the scale of the problem' (1997: 31)

The recognition of the importance of the visual domain, and specifically of television, as a 'means to message', prompted the HEA in 1990 to return to television campaigns after it had run some press-advertising-only campaigns because 'the ... absence of AIDS advertising from the small screen risks suggesting to the general public that the problem is less urgent or serious' (Field, Wellings and McVey 1997: 31). In 1999 HIV/AIDS could be described only as having been invisibilized again, since television campaigns and other major campaigns, the annual World AIDS Day 'red ribbon' sales apart, across a range of visual media were no longer run.[48] If, as Barbara Kruger (1994) puts it, 'the media partakes of a kind of "crisis construction"' (41–2), it is also instrumental in what might be termed a crisis deconstruction.[49]

The images used in the various HEA HIV prevention campaigns relied, like the ACT UP campaigns, on the verbal to convey a specific message. Indeed, as should be clear from the images shown here, without the words saying what they meant, these images might equally well have been used in mass advertising campaigns for holidays, lipstick, shampoo or perfume. Despite occupying certain kinds of visual space, the images thus relied on the word to specify the message. Indeed, if the word was not attended to, there was no HIV/AIDS-specific message in the images at all. As words made the difference in determining the meaning and conveying AIDS-specific messages in the HEA's health promotion campaigns, so words became crucial for the meaning of the art created in response to HIV/AIDS. In contrast to the health promotion campaigns which always utilized text and image and projected specific AIDS-related agendas, art work created in response to AIDS did not always work to such (specific) agendas. Nor did it always use text and image.

The art of intervention: AIDS art

In fact, the AIDS crisis produced a whole range of very different kinds of art intervention,[50] ranging, in the field of visual representation, from photodocumentary and non-realist photographic representations, memorial work such as the NAMES Project Quilt (Ruskin 1988), posters, paintings, installations to mixed-media representations, films, plays, videos and material for television, shown both in mainstream sites and outside such spaces. The very indeterminancy of the illness was reflected in the diversity of visual practices that sprang up to confront HIV/AIDS, and in the battles which ensued about questions of the most appropriate way or ways to represent HIV/AIDS.[51] The highly imaginatively constructed catalogue (Grover 1989a) of the famous

AIDS: The Artists' Response exhibition quotes Jan Zita Grover's statement: 'AIDS brings an already-existing social debate – *What is the purpose and value of art?* – to a crisis point. It throws into relief the irreducible fact that art work is based not simply (or romantically) on personal visions, but on social realities' (Grover 1989a: 35). These social realities include the fear of being ostracized by family and friends for having been identified in a film or photo documentary (see Sturrock 1993: 37; Atkins 1989: 27), the fact that some people have enough money to donate pictures by famous artists to events designed to raised money for AIDS research (Ughetto 1993) while others are homeless and suffering from AIDS, the diversities of identity among gays and lesbians (Greyson 1989), and innumerable others.

The question raised by this diversity and these social realities in the context of visual representation, 'What do we want from art in the age of AIDS?', has been answered very differently by different kinds of artists and events. In the remaining sections of this chapter I shall discuss several anti-AIDS art exhibitions from the period 1988 to 1993. These range from exhibitions curated by members of the gay community for the gay community to general art exhibitions curated for fundraising purposes. As I shall indicate, the works in the exhibitions reveal diverse positions in relation to HIV/AIDS, with some adopting strongly interventionist stances while others refuse any specific line. One key difference in this diversity resides in the use of text in or as image and images without text. In his conversation with Greg Bordowitz, Douglas Crimp[52] (1989a) said that 'it's hard to imagine how art photography can become articulate about something so complex as AIDS without the use of text' (9). I would like to re-phrase this into 'it's hard to imagine how representation can become articulate about AIDS without the use of text'. Indeed, one might argue that there is no representation of AIDS without the use of text, partly because there are so many already existent discourses on HIV/AIDS which are always already (in)directly referenced when HIV/AIDS is mentioned in any form. Additionally, art exhibitions and artists' responses are usually framed within a context where – minimally – the title of the event makes clear the connection with AIDS. But the degree of textual intervention in the visual field varies, and that variance is critical to the clarity and specificity with which HIV/AIDS is addressed.

'High' art against AIDS

The June 1993 *Drawing the Line Against AIDS*[53] exhibition, a 'high' art event, was run under the aegis of the 45th Venice Biennale at the

Peggy Guggenheim Collection to benefit the American Foundation for AIDS Research and various Italian AIDS charities.[54] Both its title and the beneficiaries of the exhibition pointed towards the connection with AIDS. The exhibition was supported by many patrons and institutions of the arts, and 'artists, art dealers and artists' estates from around the world who [had] given ... drawings' (Cheim *et al.* 1993 n.p.). While the dates of many of the drawings suggest that they were created specifically for this exhibition, this was not the case for all of them. In the knowledge of the title of the exhibition it is possible to interpret the frequently wordless *and* untitled exhibits in terms related to HIV/AIDS, though what these terms are likely to be depends very much on the viewer. Works using text directly such as Jenny Holzer's 'Untitled' (from 'The Survival Series', 1993) which states, 'In a dream you saw a way to survive/and you were full of joy', may present a specific position regarding AIDS explicitly. But this is the case with only very few of the images from this exhibition. Most of the drawings activate the reader to decide what position it and/or she or he takes *vis-à-vis* the work since they provide no textual clue as to its meaning. This allows the kind of 'purely' aesthetic contemplations that have been part of the debate of how HIV/AIDS might be represented.[55] A typical example is Günter Förg's set of four gouaches, *Untitled* (1993), which could, without difficulty, feature in any abstract art exhibition. The curators of *Drawing the Line* ... themselves assert that in the face of the horror of HIV/AIDS, 'no metaphor or allegory seems possible' (Cheim *et al.* 1993 n.p.), a position echoing Susan Sontag's (1988) resistance to metaphor in relation to AIDS.[56] The problem with that position is of course not only that all representation is *re*-presentation, therefore already at a remove from the thing itself, but also, and more importantly, that the impossibility of metaphor is asserted when a whole range of metaphors are already in circulation – Paula Treichler's (1988b) famous 'epidemic of signification' – and need to be engaged with. There is therefore no neutral ground on which horror might be encountered. The politics of the work in *Drawing the Line Against AIDS* resides, in the main, in what its viewing public makes of the work, not in the works' implicit or explicit demands or positions. One has to assume that those who supported the exhibition want to fight AIDS, and that they do so through the act of contributing rather than by the overt content of their work.

'The art of the dandy vs. the art of the activist'

This is very different from *AIDS: The Artists' Response* (1989), an exhibition grounded in the lesbian and gay communities predominantly of the USA and in particular Ohio (Grover 1989a: 5–6). Its catalogue alone defies the conventional structuring of exhibition catalogues in which articles on or statements by the artists and their work are commonly separated from representations of the work itself so that the essays occupy the opening pages of the catalogue and the representations the second part. Instead, this catalogue intersperses text and images (the latter frequently themselves including text, like Derek Jarman's AIDS canvases referred to briefly in Chapter 1), in a collage which emphasizes their interconnection and, indeed, privileges text in terms of sheer quantity. The artists' responses, which include statements about the meaning of their work, are highly articulate, politically aware and diverse, and relate the aesthetic directly to the semantic and ideological. In part the catalogue and exhibition are a testimony to the different kinds of responses artists working in diverse media have had to HIV/AIDS. Grover, the curator, stated unambiguously that 'Art addressing AIDS has more tendentious work to do than addressing modernism, postmodernism, cyberculture' (1989a: 2). *AIDS: The Artists' Response* engages with that tendentiousness directly in ways that *Drawing the Line* ... never does since work in the latter refrained – quite literally – from saying what it meant.

That tendentiousness was a source of conflicting positions among artists, especially those from the gay community. In a vehement attack on activist art and cultural activist Douglas Crimp, Richard Hawkins and Dennis Cooper (1995) described their purposes in setting up *Against Nature: A Group Show of Work by Homosexual Men*[57] as follows: 'Ingrained in "Against Nature" was a reaction against contemporary art-hating activism, the kind heralded by such critics as Douglas Crimp and entrenched in a kind of "put down your paintbrushes; this is war" production' (57). For this reason 'Prominent art collectives of the period [the late 1980s] like Testing the Limits, Group Material, Gran Fury and ACT UP were out from the beginning' (57). The show's title 'alluded to the amoral, drug-addicted aesthete anti-hero who, by engaging the anarchic powers of art, pornography and imagination, managed to distract, describe, divert and reinvest the pragmatic evils of the body' (57). This *fin de siècle* figure was also referred to by John Greyson, who exhibited both in *Against Nature* and in *AIDS: The Artists' Response*. Attempting to defend that figure, Greyson (1989) suggested that '["Against Nature"] insisted on the relevance of a particu-

lar fag sensibility in combating the AIDS crisis' (12). Greyson's video
script for 'Parma Violets' took up the debate of cultural practices
concerning AIDS, discussing 'the art of the dandy vs. the art of the
activist' (13) through the figures of Sir Richard Burton − translator of
the *Arabian Nights* and inventor of a theory of sexuality based on cli-
matic zones, − and Aschenbach, the central character of Thomas
Mann's *Death in Venice*. At one point, Sir Richard Burton is cited as
arguing that 'Just because we don't produce works that engage actual
agendas of social change doesn't mean we're ultimately vulnerable to
being recuperated by the very system we seek to disrupt' (14). One
might, of course, argue that the dandy's art, too − and this is to some
extent Hawkins and Cooper's point − engages actual agendas of social
change but does so in very particular ways, specifically through the
refusal of certain kinds of masculinity. Like ACT UP's 'Let the Record
Show …', 'Parma Violets' draws on historical precedent but in this
instance it is cultural precedent rather than a specific historical event.
Both the installation and the video expose prejudice against homosexuals and both point towards death in the current AIDS crisis, as well
as the need to respond to it. Significantly, Greyson, like those producing activist art, uses words to make his points. Textuality, or the word,
is central to his video to establish his position. The visual alone is not
enough. Tendentiousness is expressed through logocentricity.

Visualizing the invisible: positive lives

Hawkins and Cooper (1995) saw their 1988 show as a reaction against
a practice in or of art which they 'perceived as growing progressively
more pervasive, more conservative, more essentialist, more predictably
arid and photo-text based, more dependent on the conveyance of supposed hard fact and indisputable truth' (57). Yet their description of
their own show indicates that they exhibited the kinds of work they
professed to be reacting against (e.g. 'Michael Tidmus entered us into
the computer age with a 13MB display of AIDS information and
graphics' (58)). It also indicates that the work which was being produced clearly did not follow the trend they were outlining. The vari-
eties of tendentious art work from within the lesbian and gay
communities defy Hawkins and Cooper's description. As I shall discuss
below, much of the work is neither realist nor documentary in the conventional sense. Importantly, too, it foregrounds the subjective rather
than some kind of transcendent truth. The crudity of Hawkins and
Cooper's view may be juxtaposed with the work displayed in the exhibitions *Ecstatic Antibodies* (Boffin and Gupta 1990) and *Positive Lives*

(Mayes and Stein 1993). These exhibitions were UK-based and post-dated *Against Nature*. But work for these exhibitions was undertaken around the time of the *Against Nature* exhibition, and was informed by the representations of AIDS both from the USA and from the UK. It is therefore possible to draw comparisons between these exhibitions.

Positive Lives was concerned with 'Photographing the Invisible' (1993: 14), described in the accompanying book as 'the representation of a medical condition which had become a social condition'. As Mayes, one of the authors, puts it: 'many of the core subjects photographed here are invisible (feelings of love, fear, courage and alienation are no more visible than the physiological processes of a virus), but the process of photography translates these intangible miasmas into a recognizable form' (14). At the heart of the enterprise, in a sense, was the heart, not as organ but as emotion:[58] 'Documentary photography has a power to communicate with an emotional immediacy that cannot be matched by words alone' (14). For Mayes this communication depends on 'the imagination as an added ingredient', the activation of the viewer through what is seen to 'look beyond what is actually seen' (14). Mayes thus focuses on how viewers become engaged with what is presented to them, with the photo evoking the invisible through what is visible, both in terms of what it presents and in terms of how the viewer responds. However, it is the context, that is the knowledge that the exhibition is a response to HIV/AIDS as indexed through its title and the work the Terrence Higgins Trust contributed to it, as well as the texts which accompany the images, which creates the specific poignancy of the photos rather than the images alone.

The book *Positive Lives* is divided into sections which tell a sequential story, repeated through each photo sequence which also has an accompanying text-based narrative.[59] These narratives explore different positions in relation to HIV/AIDS, responding to questions such as who is affected by it and how they or we cope. However, not all images employ the grainy realism which is often associated with documentary photography. Jenny Matthews's section on 'Mothers and children' (Mayes and Stein 1993: 78–85), for instance, reflects the sense of embattlement which mothers suffering from HIV/AIDS feel and the resultant need for secrecy so as not to distress the child. The problematic of the knowledge of having HIV/AIDS, once brought out into the open, is presented literally here through an image of a can of worms (78). This concretization of a metaphor makes the invisible visible, translating emotion into an image. Other pictures by Matthews in the same section reflect the need to conceal through a focus on parts of the body rather than the whole – there are faces, cut off at various points, naked hands clasping bodies of children or concealing faces, gloved hands carrying rubbish bags, hands pressing against windows. These close-ups become evocative precisely because the closeness does not reveal the secret of the image's meaning. Intensity, focus, intimacy, all suggested by the photos, do not result in knowledge since all views are partial. These photos are not conventionally documentary in that they do not document what can be seen. Rather, they evoke what cannot be seen, they point towards the invisible.

A similar analysis might be made of the sequence 'Rupert – a life story' (Mayes and Stein 1993: 86–97). Here the focus is not on people or their non-realist representation but on environment, on places. The photographer, Paul Reas, asked Rupert, who has AIDS, to make a list of places that have been important to him, and then created photographs that reflected the atmosphere of these places. Rupert's narratives make clear that it is not the places in themselves that are significant but the experiences he associates with them. Again, this is not documentary photography in the conventional sense; reading a life through places in the way in which it is done here is not a conventional way of presenting a life story. The photographs impress first through a hand-held camera effect that presents the places from 'odd' angles, reflecting a dream-like or memory quality created through the spatial distortions which the odd angles produce. This subjectivizes the vision presented, generating the sense of a personal view, a view specific to an individual. The subjectivity of view is heightened by the fact that the places shown are glimpses or parts of views, not readily decipherable by the spectator in terms of location and meaning. In several photos it is not immediately obvious where we are or what we are seeing. Again, the viewer is activated to seek to identify the content of what is presented. Without the text and context it would not be obvious that the images have an association with HIV/AIDS.

Rupert makes the point that 'It's a curious thing, but as you approach the end of your life, ambition and future plans give way to a need to remember' (Mayes and Stein 1993: 86). The photographs thus acquire an important personal function for Rupert in externalizing the processes he is going through as part of being HIV-positive. They indicate that the audience for artistic work produced in response to HIV/AIDS is not just an uninfected, anonymous group of people but is also made up of those with HIV/AIDS, a fact not often discussed in the debates about the most appropriate way to represent AIDS. The meaning which these photographs have for Rupert is recoverable for the spectators through the accompanying text. These photographs present the invisible in a number of ways: they represent Rupert's memories, themselves invisible; they represent not just places where he has been but the experiences he associates with these places; they are a translation of the personal and private into the public.

'Art is not enough': including the other

The focus on individuals and their experiences which underlies the *Positive Lives* exhibition and structures the representations within it is radically different from the posters by a whole range of artists from different, mainly western and European countries and cultures created for the *Images pour la Lutte* ... exhibition. This exhibition of thirty-seven works was curated by Bruno Ughetto at the Centre Georges Pompidou in Paris in 1993. Of the thirty-seven works a thousand sets were made to be distributed to all kinds of public access spaces such as libraries, galleries, and schools, an educative project designed for World AIDS Day. This is not documentary art. It combines the aesthetic with the declamatory through a combination of the visual and the verbal in an effort to raise awareness. In his prefatory remarks to the exhibition (Ughetto 1993: 12) François Barré, President of the Centre Pompidou, raised the question, 'Can art, indeed, should art lend itself to a temporal struggle which by nature is locked into the limitations and bonds of service?' (Ughetto 1993: 12).[60] Barré went on to say that in a context where AIDS has led to the reversal of all our symbols, since that which is meant to give life (sex, semen) has become the instrument of death and degradation, art is important but, 'art is not enough to counter the galloping death, nor even ignominy. Only condoms will work.' While acknowledging the power of art to raise awareness, Barré also points to the limitations of art and the notion of the importance of generating awareness when he states: 'Such is the active uselessness of awareness; it is a presence to life and to death' (Ughetto 1993: 12). For Barré fighting AIDS is a matter of engaging with death. He decries the 'fractured "politically correct" awareness that breaks our whole into minorities and categories' and asserts that 'Behind the waves of leading sectorial [*sic*] thinkers ... stands a moral order of dissociation, the paradoxical loss of the significant other' (Ughetto 1993: 12). Barré's anti-factional stance is an attempt to point to the ways in which divisions such as those between the art of the dandy and the art of the activist lead to a repudiation of commonality that only the inclusion of the other can rectify. 'Every image,' he states, 'if it is just, even in its fragility, speaks to the other, to you, and to all of us' (Ughetto 1993: 12). This demand for transcendence produces a conflict with the position which asserts that AIDS is a series of epidemics rather than one, and that individual needs differ and therefore need to be differentially addressed. Barré's statements stem from a time (1993), however, when certain images associated with AIDS such as the equation of homosexuality with AIDS, or death with AIDS, were already well entrenched,[61] were indeed one reason why this exhibition was held. He thus articulates a position intended to counter the kinds of prejudices activist art too sought to fight.

The images presented in *Images* ... reflect a range of attitudes towards HIV/AIDS. Images without words such as the black-and-white candle burning at both ends (75), an ostrich looking alertly at the camera (57), or a drawing of a pear from which a worm emerges about to crawl into an apple which already has a hole (24), could be read as forms of condemnation – but of whom? Those infected with HIV? Those avoiding engagement with the epidemic? Others, such as Paris-Clavel's drawing of male genitals in the form of a pistol with the words 'Don't forget the condom – thank you' inscribed on the image, play upon the dominant message of the period about the importance of condom use for HIV prevention. Roger Pfund's 'Isolé' simultaneously explores a private experience and a public response to AIDS. Pfund's image has as its background a kaleidescopic photograph of a crowd, with the off-centre focus bringing into relief a small group of people. This crowd is juxtaposed with a small copy of a page from a passport in the bottom right-hand corner. This page has two stars stamped into it and shows, in sharp relief, a passport photo of a bearded man. Across the whole image, from the bottom left-hand corner to the top right-hand one, the word 'Isolé' (Isolated) is stamped. The image both suggests the loneliness someone with HIV/AIDS may experience and points to the idea, notoriously expressed in the USA by Senator William F. Buckley Jr, that people with AIDS should be branded as such by having a tattoo imprinted on their private parts (Miller 1993: 215).[62] *Images* ... for the most part contains images that utilize text to make their point, which verbalize their message. The messages address both personal and public agendas, exposing the tension between the two.

Conclusion

In the fight for the words to say it, to name, define and intervene in relation to HIV/AIDS, different types of cultural production, driven by the agendas of their originators, produced diverse and often contradictory messages. These messages were created predominantly at the level of the word, since the images utilized in themselves often did not convey a specific HIV/AIDS agenda. Words thus became indispensible to HIV/AIDS prevention and intervention work. The visibilization of HIV/AIDS issues relied on words as the prime instrument for creating cultural space to intervene in the advance of HIV/AIDS. However, this cultural space was imbued with contradictions which served to reinforce the cultural separatism that had generated the scapegoating of gays in the first few years of the HIV/AIDS epidemic. Non-specificity, as much as inappropriate singling out of certain groups of people, contributed to this and made people of colour, to use a US term, already 'other' in western culture, one of the groups further alienated through the process of visibilizing AIDS. This is the focus of the following chapter as it considers attempts to locate HIV/AIDS through various forms of mapping.

Notes

1 *The Words to Say It* is the title of a novel by Marie Cardinal (1975) in which she details how the ability to name what troubles her saves a woman from the permanent menstruating from which she suffers as the consequence of her not having 'the words to say it'.

2 The health promotion campaigns utilized media such as television, poster campaigns and the press to address their audiences, thus reaching a wide and more diffuse audience whereas much of the art work was displayed in gallery sites, and therefore reached not only much smaller audiences but also those audiences specifically inclined to visit galleries and museums.

3 Strictly speaking, images without text occur rarely since the contexts in which they are displayed often have a word-based title; even images without text often either have specific titles or are 'untitled'.

4 For an interesting discussion of the difficulties faced by the HEA in its own relationship with the Department of Health over HIV/AIDS representation in the public domain see Miller and Williams (1993).

5 See Watney (1997) and Scott (1997) for a critique of the implicit attitudes towards the gay community and gay AIDS activism expressed through these campaigns.

6 In 1990 the Swiss health authorities for example ran a series of ads trying to counter ignorance about how one might 'catch' AIDS. The captions were in the form of brief statements such as 'Mosquitoes. No risk of AIDS'; 'Petting. No risk of AIDS'; 'Kissing. No risk of AIDS'; 'Exchanging glasses. No risk of AIDS.'; 'Sneezing, coughing. No risk of AIDS'.

7 Thus in 1990 *The Guardian* reported the case of an 'Aids-snub nurse dropped' about a nurse struck off the nursing register for refusing to care for patients with AIDS, HIV and hepatitis.

8 See, for instance, Watney (1994: 25; 1987: 1); Roxan (1984); O'Flaherty (1983).

9 The gay community as an authority was ignored.

10 For a brief critique of the abstraction of the early HEA anti-AIDS campaigns see Watney (1994: 19–21).

11 The non-specificity of the notion that everybody is potentially at risk and may become HIV-positive has been the object of much subsequent critique, particularly from gay men who consider this position to have contributed significantly to the de-

gaying of AIDS-campaigns (e.g. Bronski 1997; Odets 1997).

12 The campaign completely ignored women's experience of their safety as frequently not a matter of their choice.

13 Another poster featured the text 'TWO EYES NOSE MOUTH', with the words positioned to form these features as if on a face. The text underneath the black block read, 'How to recognise someone with HIV ...'. The implied message here was that anybody could be a carrier.

14 For a discussion of the impact of this message on HIV-positive men see Grimshaw (1989: 214ff).

15 Other campaigns, sometimes in very sinister fashion, also played on the notion of voluntarism. In 1990 the AIDS Action Council in the USA, for instance, ran a white-on-black campaign which stated: 'You don't just catch AIDS. You have to let somebody give it to you.'

16 For an extended discussion of the new right discourse of the 1980s see Smith (1994).

17 This line completely failed to take into account any power differentials between men and women in determining their own 'safety' within a sexual context. See Richardson (1994a: 51–2) and Holland et al. (1994a) for a critique of this failure.

18 This contradicts Waldby's (1996) emphatic assertion that the social order made visible by the struggles around AIDS management presents the heterosexual masculine as human and normal and 'largely unmarked by a "risk" status within the epidemic' (9–10). Indeed, there is worldwide evidence to the contrary; the Ministry of Health in Zimbabwe, for example, ran a poster campaign before 1990 which featured a man talking to a woman saying, 'AIDS Kills: What ... will you take home with you? Make sure it's not AIDS' (AID-CH: n.p.) where the addressee, that is the person perceived to be at risk, was clearly a heterosexually active male. Switzerland ran a series of campaigns which had text in different handwriting, signalling diverse individuals, that stated 'I don't use condoms because ...' which were then commented on in terms of their truth-value and/or appropriateness as a position. At least three of these posters centred on heterosexually active men, with statements such as 'I don't use condoms because I'm not gay'; 'I don't use condoms because women don't like them'; and 'I don't use condoms because they reduce sensation' (AID-CH: n.p.).

19 It is important to note that fear related to sex for women is multiple, associated with the possibility of violence from a man, with getting pregnant and with being stigmatized as a 'slut'. In addition, and specifically in relation to the timing of this campaign, it has to be remembered that particularly in the late 1980s in the UK, the memory of the Yorkshire Ripper, an emblem of a man attacking and killing women within a sexualized context, was still strong (see Cameron and Frazer 1987).

20 Text reproduced by kind permission of the Health Education Authority.

21 This is indicative of Wilton's (1994) point that 'HIV/AIDS health promotion has failed to identify and engage with the interaction between the social construction of gender and the social construction of sexuality ... which differentially constitute feminine and masculine sexual subjectivity' (85).

22 For a discussion of the representation of inarticulacy in sexual situations as represented in both heterosexual and lesbian pulp (romance) fiction see Griffin (1995: 145–8).

23 The issue of the unspoken in homosexual encounters was paradoxically and contradictorily raised in two campaigns aimed at gay men publicized in Germany in 1989. One, a poster showing two gay men, one semi-nude, the other in leather with an arm around the first man, said: 'Ohne viele Worte. Alles was geil und sicher ist – Safer Sex' ('Without having to talk about it. Anything that is sexy and safe – Safer Sex'). The other, also a poster aimed at gay men, showed two men in a café or bar together with the caption: 'Lokalkolorit. Quatschen, Klatschen, Freunde treffen. Über alles reden. Auch über Sex. Sicher' ('Local colour. Chatting, gossiping, meeting friends.

Talk about everything. About sex too. Safe[ly]'). Thus whilst one poster in the context of an implied imminent sexual moment suggested that one did *not* have to talk but could take certain things such as only indulging in safer sex practices for granted, the other stated that in a wider social setting one might want to talk about everything including safer sex (practices) as part of one's ordinary everyday conversations. Perhaps the assumption was that having cleared the ground, so to speak, at the café, no further discussion about what sexual practices and precautions to engage in was necessary during a sexual encounter.

24 There is a correlation between the notion of sex existing within the realm of the unarticulated and the notion that, as Gilman (1997) puts it, 'that which is hidden is that which is eroticized' (110).

25 When the romance fiction publisher Mills & Boon first introduced condom use into its novels in recognition of the AIDS threat, clear gendered lines were drawn: the man constructed as the active and knowing partner provided the condom and knew what it was, 'tactfully' turning aside while he put it on; the woman, passive and sexually innocent, seemed totally ignorant of condoms.

26 See, for example, Holland *et al.* (1996) and DeHardt (1993) for discussions of the unequal power structures which inform heterosexual relationships and sex-related decision-making within these.

27 Silk Cut and Benson & Hedges advertisements are obvious examples here.

28 In discussing the relationship between health-related (drinking; smoking) and sexual behaviour, Wellings *et al.* (1994) unsurprisingly report that 'there is a relationship between a number of risk-taking behaviours' (292).

29 See Douglas (1966) for an extended analysis of the ways in which fear and blame operate as part of the way in which taboos are culturally managed.

30 The use of images of women in the context of discussions and representations of sexually transmitted diseases has been widely discussed (see, for example, Gilman 1988a; Park 1993).

31 Waldby (1996) analyses the use of militaristic vocabulary in the context of AIDS.

32 For critiques of the notion that 'everybody is at risk' see Oppenheimer and Reckitt (1997).

33 Such notions of agency play to both a particularly masculinized version of the sense of self as subject and also to a very middle-class idea of how individuals perceive themselves.

34 The first HEA campaigns ran in 1986–7; they thus postdated the death from AIDS of Rock Hudson, for instance (Kinsella 1989), pictures of whom from both before and after the onset of AIDS had widely circulated in the world press. The recognition of the homosexuality of this Hollywood (hetero)sex symbol was one of the many ways in which a sense of people's 'ignorance' about sexuality was reinforced in reactions to the AIDS crisis, then to be expressed as such in the 'Don't Die of Ignorance' campaign.

35 A good example of this is charity advertising for charities dealing with disability. The explicit aestheticization of bodies in advertisements of the Multiple Sclerosis Society run in the UK in the mid-1990s for example vividly emphasized the non-admissability of the ill body within cultural mainstream sites such as advertising hoardings on the Underground.

36 Crimp (1997), for example, poignantly highlights this when he states his concern about 'ageing as a gay man, for which there is little or no discourse at all. The older gay man doesn't exist in gay culture, except as a couple of horrible stereotypes – the dirty old man, the sad old queen. The founding moment of psychoanalysis in the shift away from the visibility of the hysteric has its parallel in relation to homosexuality … One of the things the older gay man does in order to maintain any sort of position in gay culture is to don a uniform. There's a stereotype about the leather

scene, that's where we end up when we get older' (Iversen, Crimp and Bhabha 1997: 20–1, 24).

37 It is important to acknowledge that the kind of decision-making implied in many of the AIDS prevention campaigns do not reflect the realities of interactions in sexual encounters.

38 Bronski (1997) makes clear: 'Ironically, safer sex campaigns which avoided depicting bodies with visible signs of AIDS did so, in part, to avoid stigmatizing people with AIDS, to present positive and negative alike as beautiful' (123–4).

39 The photo evokes a multiplicity of associations from the Greek figure of Tiresias to the so-called Elephant Man. Its beauty or 'classical austerity' is thus a function of its ability to signal 'transcendence'.

40 In an unpublished article (personal communication to the author) Richard Sawdon Smith discusses the reception of his prize-winning photo and quotation from correspondence he had with the editor of *The Times*, and from correspondence in *Amateur Photographer*, which published the picture. Peter Stothard, the editor, is quoted as stating that 'If it was of any importance to the judges that *The Times* publish the winning photograph, it would have been prudent of them to give some discussion to its acceptability'.

41 In an interesting chapter, Laura Mulvey (1973) shows how the issue of the portrayal of male genitals translates into the fetishization of the female body.

42 Vance (1994) makes the point that 'though we may reject the overly literal connection that conservatives like to make between images and action ... we know too that diversity in images and expression in the public sector nurtures and sustains diversity in private life. When losses are suffered in public arenas, people for whom controversial or minority images are salient and affirming suffer a real defeat. Defending private rights – to behaviour, to images, to information – is difficult without a publicly formed and visible community' (99).

43 For a discussion of the changes in representation of the condom as a consequence of the AIDS epidemic see Treichler (1997).

44 Feminist critiques of these campaigns (Kitzinger 1994; Wilton 1994; Richardson 1994a) have pointed out the absence of information about non-penetrative forms of sex which are safer for women than penetrative intercourse.

45 A *Guardian* report in 1990 on a then new Kinsey sex survey stated that most respondents (men and women, mostly heterosexual) 'use oil-based lubricants like petroleum jelly with a condom, even though 60 seconds of intercourse will then produce microscopic holes through which the AIDS virus can pass, and another 40 seconds produces holes through which sperm can pass' (Walker 1990).

46 Kitzinger (1994) and Richardson (1994b) have pointed out that lesbians' needs remain unaddressed in all of these campaigns.

47 Wilton (1994) discusses the problematic of the eroticization of health promotion campaign material where conflicting discourses collide.

48 World AIDS Day (1 December) and the red ribbon continue, but the continual presence of the red ribbon has normalized that symbol into a sign whose significance is as a reminder of 'AIDS' but without any form of direct address or message. Its efficacy is in the notion of the non-specific reminder, in maintaining a non-specific awareness level.

49 'De-construction' is here used in its commonsensical meaning rather than as a specific theoretical term.

50 One text examining this range is Ted Gott's *Don't Leave Me This Way: Art in the Age of AIDS* (1994).

51 See, for example, Hawkins and Cooper (1995); Crimp (1989a); Greyson (1989); Watney (1989a).

52 Bordowitz was consistently more moderate in his line than Crimp. This is, however, emphatically not a critique of Crimp's position, which I think has frequently been misunderstood.

53 Since the catalogue is not paginated but work pictured is ordered alphabetically by the artists' surnames, I shall refer to their names when commenting on individual works.

54 This exhibition followed on from the first international *Art Against AIDS* exhibition held in Basel, Switzerland, in 1991.

55 See, for example, Hawkins and Cooper (1995); Miller (1993); Crimp (1989a); Sontag (1988).

56 Sontag's position has been severely critiqued, by Miller (1993) among others.

57 This show ran January to February 1988 at LACE (Los Angeles Contemporary Exhibitions).

58 It is worth noting that many of the introductions to exhibitions from the late 1980s and early 1990s played on the notion of emotion and evoking emotional responses in artists and viewers. François Barré, President of the Centre Pompidou in Paris, said, for example, that 'art is the expression, among others, of love and freedom [which] are precisely what AIDS is questioning and killing' (Ughetto 1993: 12). Hence the need, in his view, for the *Images* ... exhibition. Emotion seemed to become the key to dealing with the invisible.

59 For a brief discussion about the need to disrupt the narrative conventions of crisis and resolution which inform dominant representations of HIV/AIDS see Selden (1993).

60 This question compares interestingly with many gay artists' assertion that in the time of AIDS they find it impossible to work on anything not associated with that disease.

61 Several of the exhibitions of this period focused powerfully on death. In his foreword to *Positive Lives* Edmund White, for instance, himself HIV-positive and then with a lover who had AIDS, wrote: 'The person with AIDS ... sees through necessity to the end of all needs – death. This vision neutralizes everything that is cosy, familiar and automatic. Someone once said that we couldn't go on living if we knew the moment of our death. AIDS gives us that tragic certainty' (Mayes and Stein 1993: 7).

62 It also points to the Holocaust and the branding of Jews and homosexuals through marks of difference.

4

Locations: mapping HIV/AIDS in Randy Shilts's *And the Band Played On* and other texts

'We could be due for another killer as all-pervasive as the plague.'

'Where would it come from? Outer space?'

'Who knows. It could be hibernating in some unexplored corner of the earth, some fragment of primitive forest, and carried by a creature so small, no one has noticed it.'

'A new virus?'

'Not necessarily a virus, but probably: a disease as contagious as small-pox, as virulent as plague, coming newly into a world without inherited immunity and no present knowledge. It would take time to isolate. Before being isolated, it could bring human numbers down at a very satisfactory speed.' (Manning 1974: 162)

Both of us are getting worse
Neither knows who had it first

He thinks I gave it to him
I think he gave it to me

(Kay 1991: 50)

The conversation from Olivia Manning's 1974 novel *The Rainforest* reproduced above may seem to some uncannily prophetic of stories of the emergence of the HIV virus as circulated in medical and other *narratives* of the 1980s. Its uncanniness, however, resides not in its resemblance to what actually occurred, that is any 'real' history of the HIV virus, but in its similarity to, or reiteration of, narratives about the HIV virus which were written a decade or more after Manning's novel. Its uncanniness is therefore a function of the repetition of certain stories recurrently told in western culture, while the lines from Kay's poem, also quoted above, reflect the state of ignorance we are really in concerning the origin of HIV/AIDS.

In Manning's novel the prospective killer virus is defined along three co-ordinates: as a 'creature' co-existing with another, a living organism of a kind, itself whole and separate from others; as geographically determinate though remote (coming from outer space, some unexplored corner of the earth or some fragment of 'primitive' forest); and as present but not yet manifest. It is a matter of time and opportunity before the latter will occur. In the novel, a discredited European doctor, one of the speakers in this conversation, leads a fellow Englishman, also down at heel, to a remote and forbidden part of an island off West Africa, where, indeed, the virus appears to reside, hosted by a spider. The doctor, hitherto immune to the bite of the spider, succumbs and dies, leaving the Englishman to find his way back out of the remote part of the island, with the state of his own health uncertain. This context for the conversation between the doctor and the Englishman indicates a narrative expressive of a specific history of representations of the relationship between Europe and Africa which is part of the social imaginary of colonial powers in decline. Unable to imagine themselves as the source of disease, they figure the virus as 'crafty little creatures constantly trying to outsmart humans in their bid for survival' (Shilts 1987: 73),[1] residing in spaces which are uninhabitable from a European perspective and which are 'out there' as opposed to 'right here'. Sandra Harding (1998) has emphasized the eurocentricity of western science which is concerned with understanding illnesses affecting Europeans or Caucasians, and regarding them as emanating from 'foreign' countries, whilst using other and 'othered' countries as laboratories for the development of their science. This phenomenon can in some respects be observed in relation to HIV/AIDS, the origins of which remain debated.[2] The problematic of the invisibility of HIV/AIDS is thus reinforced by uncertainty about its/their origins which continues to be a matter of discussion nearly two decades into the knowledge of the existence of HIV/AIDS.

In this chapter I want to analyse what lies behind the continued attempts to locate the origins of the HIV virus. I shall discuss three examples of how the uncertainty about the origins of HIV and AIDS has manifested itself in the history of their representation in order to raise questions about how the 'failure' to attribute HIV/AIDS unambiguously to a specifiable materiality has impacted on the representation of HIV and AIDS. The examples – the debates about the relationship between HIV and AIDS; Randy Shilts's (1987) *And the Band Played On*; and a set of 'Pass notes on AIDS' from *The Guardian* (1993) – reflect three questions raised again and again in relation to HIV/AIDS:

• Is HIV the cause of AIDS or not?

- Where does it come from?
- Whose fault is it?[3]

HIV and AIDS: a causal relationship

Although it is now widely accepted that AIDS does not exist without HIV infection, this view is not entirely without critics. Even in 1999, with millions of pounds and dollars spent on discovering ways of treating HIV infection and AIDS-related illnesses, dissident voices promoting a different view still appear.[4] In April 1999 the *Times Higher Educational Supplement* (*THES*) carried an article in its 'Features' section about Kary Mullis, an American Nobel Prize winner who maintained that 'he cannot find any research to support the notion that HIV is the probable cause of Aids' (Ochert 1999). About a month later the *THES* then published two follow-up pieces: an article by Gordon Stewart, emeritus professor of public health at the University of Glasgow, and a letter by Britain's foremost AIDS activist and writer, Simon Watney. Stewart produced a history of the controversy over whether HIV causes AIDS or not. The key issue is that there has been no *confirmation by isolation* of the original retrovirus, so that the presence of antibodies has been used as the confirmatory sign of the presence of the virus. 'Proof positive' so to speak is, in Stewart's view, still missing.

The underlying assumption, that only the confirmation by isolation or actual presence of the virus can prove its existence and its causal relation to AIDS, reflects the positivist attitude governing western science. When I went to visit a Chinese herbalist some years ago and asked him how what he had prescribed me (tea made up of a variety of ingredients) would 'work', he told me that the notion of isolating a specific element or ingredient and then replicating it artificially was a typically western way of identifying diseases and treatments – he mentioned penicillin as an example. He said that he could not tell me how and why the tea would work since – though he had studied medicine in China – the knowledge that it would work was a matter of experience[5] accumulated over two thousand years in Chinese medicine and passed on through Chinese medical education. The tea worked. The conversation highlighted the ethnocentricity of western medicine, driven by particular notions of cause and effect, and by the idea of singling out, visibilizing in atomistic fashion, a part which will, or is supposed to, make sense of the whole. Similarly, the debate about whether or not HIV causes AIDS is driven by the desire for a confirmation along the lines of cause and effect which, in its narrowest sense, leads people like Gordon Stewart to raise questions about the reliability of asserting HIV as cause and AIDS as effect.

Stewart (1999) maintains that 'With the "discovery" of HIV, the universally infectious retrovirus, and the conversion of this hypothesis into a dogma, all dissent began to be suppressed'. He is not alone in his critique of the assertion of a causal relationship between HIV and AIDS.[6] In his article he points to Professor Peter Duesberg[7] who, in 1987, suggested that 'HIV was a latent virus incapable of causing AIDS'. Duesberg has his own website where he publicizes his work and so-called dissident voices, including that of journalist John Lauritsen, who on the 'Rethinking AIDS home page' publishes 'Looking back on Berlin', an account of events which occurred at the 9th International AIDS conference in Berlin in 1993. There, as Lauritsen puts it, 'for the first time at an international AIDS conference, alternative voices could be heard, attacking the HIV-hypothesis, anti-viral therapy, and other AIDS dogmas'. These alternative voices were, according to Lauritsen, counter-attacked: 'the AIDS Empire struck back'. Lauritsen concludes that international AIDS conferences are 'trade shows. Their entire purpose is to promote the commodities of the AIDS Industry. They are about buying and selling.' This is not dissimilar to the line taken by Stewart, who maintains that 'Secretive censorship is familiar to anyone who has questioned orthodox views on Aids ... There are, naturally, vested interests involved: many individuals receive high rewards for their work within orthodox Aids science ... the pharmaceutical companies have their own agenda.'

The language employed by Lauritsen and in the article on Kary Mullis (Ochert 1999) deserves some attention. Drawing on the discourses employed to discuss voices who took an oppositional stance in what used to be communist regimes but who are or were approved of by the west, they speak of the AIDS establishment and an AIDS orthodoxy (which seems perilously close to a fundamentalist position, and is ironic given the 'outsider' status accorded to groups like ACT UP) underwritten by multinational pharmaceutical companies (the cynicism of capitalism) against which these 'dissidents' – legitimate voices driven underground – attempt to assert themselves. The Internet becomes the space in which that voice can manifest itself, as a visualized presence on websites, visibilizing its 'dissent' in a space which escapes regulation and, as Lauritsen puts it, 'the brutal disregard which was shown for the principle of free enquiry' (1993) at the Berlin conference. The outer space of the Internet is complemented by the reference to the empire striking back – a fight at once medieval, colonial, dualist, high-tech and fictional. The appropriation of the term 'dissident' (and it is ironic that several of the most prominent dissidents from the former communist states in eastern Europe were, after the collapse of those states, shown to have collaborated closely with the secret services of their respective countries) serves to legitimate a stance which has incensed many of those at the forefront of fighting HIV/AIDS in the west such as AIDS activist groups, and which has been met with sustained scepticism by the majority of the medical establishment. Indeed, the *THES* in 1995 printed a UK news item which stated, as the headline put it, 'HIV link confirmed' and detailed that a fifteen-year study of haemophiliacs by the Medical Research Council had proved 'conclusively that HIV is the cause of AIDS'. The point is that the state of knowledge, frequently represented as epistemic certainty, keeps changing and that this movement does not follow a linear structure as the history of science would sometimes have it. In his 1999 letter to the *THES* condemning Kary Mullis's stance on HIV/AIDS, Simon Watney maintained: 'The clinical association between HIV and AIDS has been irrefutably demonstrated in count-less epidemiological surveys since the late 1980s. In a nutshell, where there is no HIV, there is no AIDS.' Significantly, Watney talks of *asso-ciation* rather than cause and effect. He thus circumvents the linearity which informs other positions. The diverse terminologies employed by the different factions in the debates about the relationship between HIV and AIDS index the uncertainty about the precise nature of that relationship. Since the virus itself has not been 'confirmed by isolation', its presence has to be discerned through another presence, that of the antibodies. These can be made visible through various tests and ampli-fications. But they are effectively second-order presences, pointing to the absence of the proof positive of the virus itself. The contestation of the virus's presence is indicative of the need for visible signs, 'seeing is believing', for the visibility of the 'thing-itself' within the discourse of western science. Simultaneously, the debates about the relationship between HIV and AIDS are a measure of the discursive dependency which this uncertainty gives rise to: the words in which you say it become everything.[8] Textual contestation and textual debates take the place of the visible sign which is lacking. The resultant textualization draws the various narratives which are produced into the conventions which govern the forms chosen for the textual actualization of the quest for the origin of HIV and AIDS.

Tracking HIV/AIDS

This is very evident in Randy Shilts's (1987) 'ground-breaking book' and now 'major tv movie' as the cover of my copy puts it, *And the Band Played On*. In the 'Notes on sources' the book is described as 'a work of journalism. There has been no fictionalization' (623). But the subsequent discussion of 'narrative flow' points to a concern with storytelling predominantly associated with literary, indeed fictional, modes. The reference to 'the people who play a key role in this book' (623) alludes to another cultural form, that of the theatre, replicated at the beginning of the text by a list of 'Dramatis personae'. These are the people who play the key roles in Shilts's text. They have both a real-life presence, that is exist in the material world, and simultaneously become characters in Shilts's narrative. The status of that narrative, poised among different forms of textual construction (journalism, play, fiction, documentary), thus acquires an ambiguity which is, however, ultimately not shared by the content of the narrative since the latter is driven by realist conventions which suggest narrative linearity and promote closure. Of the realist conventions employed, the key ones are the use of dramatis personae who represent 'real' people, and the reference to chronological time and spaces which have their counterparts in the material world. The effects generated by these realist conventions will be discussed below.

And the Band ... seeks to create a particular narrative of HIV/AIDS. Its mock-apocalyptic section headings, reminiscent of the drawings of Francisco de Goya, of which the most obvious ones are 'Behold, a pale horse', 'The gathering darkness', 'Battle lines' and 'The butcher's bill', reflect the sense of doom surrounding HIV/AIDS felt by many in the second half of the 1980s, the time when this book was written. In keeping with the quasi-mythological images of war invoked through the section headings which suggest the devastation and butchery of a war in which men are cut to pieces, the text of *And the Band* ... is divided up into segments. These segments are not randomized, however; they only seemingly generate an image of fragmentation for they are structured through two devices: chronology and geography, time and space. These vectors serve as co-ordinates in a grid, the purpose of which is to trace HIV/AIDS, to map its occurence rather as one might chart a journey. It generates two effects: a 'reality effect' as Roland Barthes (1986b) describes it through the referencing of particular times and places which we recognize as having counterparts in material reality as we know it, *and* the sense that the local is connected to the global through the sequentiality and simultaneity which characterize time and space. The initially seemingly unconnected locations juxtaposed in the narrative, which moves from New York Harbour to Kinshasa, Zaïre, to Hjardemaal, Denmark in the first chapter alone, will, in the course of the text, make sense as parts of a story whose local manifestations fit within a globally significant phenomenon. Shilts's story thus takes on the characteristics of a map (he talks of a 'biological landscape' (1987: xxi)) on which a movement is charted, pinpointing particular locations and gradually making connections among these which are intended, in turn, to bring into focus the meaning and, indeed, resolution of his narrative. For, bounded as his story is by the conventions of realism as indexed in the use of particular time-space co-ordinates, its narrative structure bears the citational traces of realist fiction, or naturalist drama, with a (mysterious and mystifying) beginning, complicating (and complicated) middle, and an end or resolution. Within this structure, time and space are used as ways of marking or making visible the traces of the phenomenon Shilts seeks to map – HIV/AIDS.

Shilts's attempt at charting or visibilizing HIV/AIDS takes the form of a medico-cultural geography. The map which Shilts produces suggests movement or a journey. The notion of the journey is a significant metaphor here since it evokes the idea of migrancy and mobility as well as the notion of temporary presence or visibility. For journeys are about temporary presences. Such temporary presences are suggested in the first section of the text, which begins with a scene in New York Harbour. The harbour itself is, of course, simultaneously an image of a haven, a place of security, safety and permanence, *and* an image of migrancy and temporality since, as the first two paragraphs repeatedly make clear, 'ships from fifty-five nations had poured sailors into Manhattan' and 'the guests had come from all over the world' (3). This movement from the outside in, similar to the acquisition of a virus (or invasion of the host by foreign bodies), sets the scene for one of the movements described throughout the text, that of the invasion of North America, a hospitable (ironic word here!) nation, by HIV/AIDS to which, for a long time, it played unsuspecting host. Summing up the opening scene of *And the Band ...* in New York Harbour on 4 July 1976 which 'hosted the greatest party ever known', Shilts writes: 'This was the part the epidemiologists would later note, when they stayed up late at night and the conversation drifted toward where it had started and when' (3). Significantly, not Shilts but medical experts are interpellated as the ones who make the connections which Shilts, by implication, only reports. Shilts deflects his narrative presence on to these experts, using the device of the omniscient narrator who can look ahead into the future from a privileged position of knowledge as a way of authenticating the position and location he adopts in the time before the future – the experts will come to see as significant what he, presciently, has already declared as such from a position of hindsight recast as foresight. The device of the omniscient narrator, a stock-in-trade of realist fiction, makes possible the projection of the prospect of closure, of a notion that everything is knowable and known and can therefore, ultimately, be resolved. Against the uncertainty of the origins of HIV/AIDS, a narrative is thus set up which projects certainty.

In Shilts's narrative, the counterpart to the unwitting hosting of a great party in New York Harbour and its after-effects is the benign presence in Kinshasa, Zaïre, of European and American doctors, sent for, according to Shilts's story, by 'frightened African health officials' who had 'swallowed their pride' in the face of 'a virulent outbreak of a horrifiying new disease' and had 'called the World Health Organiza-tion, who came with a staff from the American Centers for Disease Control' (4). Unlike the American scenario detailed above, in which the American nation plays unwitting host to invading foreign bodies, here the Americans and Europeans are constructed not as foreign bodies invading Africa but as helpers invited in and come to support those in need while at the same time, heroically and selflessly, putting them-selves and their own lives at risk since 'The lack of rudimentary sup-plies meant that a surgeon's work had risks that doctors in the developed world could not imagine, particularly because the undevel-oped part, specifically Central Africa, seemed to sire new diseases with nightmarish regularity' (4). Shilts sets up his story by juxtaposing two locations, recreating an opposition between the developed and the undeveloped world which will serve both to locate, and to form the basis of, certain judgements already implicit in the construction of for-eigners versus Americans and Europeans. The knowledge claims made in this text are, as Lorraine Code (1995) describes it, 'invested claims' (71), reproducing particular standpoints which the reader is invited to share. The very success of the book ('now a major tv movie') is indica-tive of the kind of standpoint reproduced, one where America plays host to, but is not the origin of, foreign bodies which are, in this nar-rative, 'sired' by Africa.[9] America thus becomes a victim of foreign bodies not of its making.

This is reinforced through the specificity of the key figure which Shilts introduces into his narrative: Gaitan Dugas, also known as Patient Zero.[10] This figure mirrors the structural device of the mapping and charting of a journey utilized by Shilts: Gaitan Dugas is an airline steward – his very profession an index of his migrancy, his mobility, the temporality of his presence, and his un-site-ability. He is nowhere and everywhere, transmogrifying into a myth precisely because of his un-locatability. But he also comes from elsewhere, like the guests in New York Harbour 'all the way from …' – in this case, Toronto (11).

At the beginning of the story he is not a resident of North America – he is Canadian and, what is more, from the French-speaking part of Canada. His non-Americanness, and the identity of an assumed key carrier and spreader of the HIV virus as being non-American, is thus fully realized. He is an other whose otherness is multiply marked through his migrancy, his homosexuality and through the exotic attraction which he exudes: 'He bought his clothes in the trendiest shops of Paris and London. He vacationed in Mexico and on the Caribbean beaches. Americans tumbled for his soft Québecois accent and his sensual magnetism. There was no place that the twenty-eight-year-old airline steward would rather have the boys fall for him than in San Francisco' (21). Gaitan Dugas emerges as the itinerant seducer of unsuspecting American boys who fall for his exotic charms. His foreignness and his sensuality replicate standard tropes of 'the other' as projected in colonial narratives and consistently critiqued in postcolonial theory.[11] Shilts attributes pivotal significance to this figure in his narrative: 'Later, when researchers started referring to Gaetan Dugas simply as Patient Zero, they would retrace the airline steward's travels during that summer, fingering through his fabric-covered address book to try to fathom the bizarre coincidences and the unique role the handsome young steward performed in the coming epidemic' (23). It is, in a sense, through this figure that Shilts invites the reader to make sense of his narrative which begins to form into a very particular kind of story, a story with heroes and villains, perpetrators and victims, others and selves. And, as indicated above, it is not Shilts but 'experts' or researchers who are constructed as putting together the narrative which Shilts has unravelled for the reader, only to re-assemble it into the coherent whole he keeps promising the reader and of which the various experts he invokes become the guarantors.

Central to this story is the notion of the foreigner who infects unsuspecting victims with the virus he carries. The foreignness of HIV/AIDS is stressed again and again: it is 'elderly Jewish or Italian men' who get Kaposi's sarcoma (20), one of the symptoms of AIDS. Prior to that, 'in 1914, Kaposi's sarcoma, or KS, was first reported in Africa, where subsequent studies discovered that it was the most common tumor found among the Bantus, the disease generally remaining within distinct geographic boundaries in the open savannah of central Africa' (37). In Shilts's narrative, Africa emerges as the breeding ground of 'the killer that quietly stalked three continents in the 1980s': 'a new virus was now well-entrenched on three continents, having moved easily from Africa to Europe and then to North America' (49). As Treichler (1989) puts it, 'The Third World typically enters the First World discourse more or less unconsciously as a stereotypically reliable explanatory figure for the exotic and the alien' (32). Shilts's chain of evidence provides a linear and sequential narrative which constructs North America as the victim of something which did not originate on its soil. Location becomes the key to the mystery which is generated through the movement of its protagonists and specifically, but not exclusively, through the movements of Gaetan Dugas, who features as the emblem and the epicentre of how HIV/AIDS in North America happened.

The mapping exercise which Shilts undertakes is mirrored in his narrative by another mapping – done by one of the experts Shilts constructs to authenticate his text. In representing the work of William Darrow, a 'sociologist and epidemiologist involved with AIDS research at the Centers for Disease Control' (1987: xiii), Shilts generates a map within a map (his own narrative) when he writes: 'By the time Bill Darrow's research was done, he had established sexual links between 40 patients in ten cities. At the center of the cluster diagram was Gaetan Dugas, marked on the chart as Patient Zero of the GRID epidemic ... The Los Angeles Cluster Study, as it became known, offered powerful evidence that GRID not only was transmitted but was the work of a single infectious agent' (147). Shilts's map of geographical locations is thus overlaid with a sociogram which maps the connections among individuals, visibilizing connections and tracking movements. Shilts describes the effect of this on one man, Dr Marcus Conant, another of Shilts's dramatis personae who, on hearing about the cluster study, 'immediately recognized Patient Zero as the suave Québecois airline steward who had come into his office the month before. He was the type of man everyone wanted. What everyone had wanted was bringing them death' (155).

At the centre of the narrative is the locatability of Patient Zero – an individual who can be held responsible for the spread of the HIV virus. Cast as a roving figure of death, Gaetan Dugas becomes one of the scapegoats in Shilts's text, which states that owing to 'the popularity of air travel ... it took just one person here or there to carry the right virus to the right population, and disease would strike again' (156–7). The attribution of guilt to a single figure – a device commonly employed in detective and crime fiction but also, of course, in Christian mythology – generates expiatory opportunities as a reward for tracking down that guilty person. Shilts reinforces the notion of Dugas's guilt by reproducing 'rumors of a strange guy ... a blond with a French accent ... [who] would have sex with you, turn up the lights in the cubicle, and point out his Kaposi's sarcoma lesions. "I've got gay cancer," he'd say. "I'm going to die and so are you"' (165). Dugas is constructed as the prototype of the person who, once aware of his illness, passes it on deliberately as a way of retaliating for having become infected in the first instance.[12]

And the Band ... does not directly answer the question where or how Dugas became infected. His infection is linked to his itineracy, and to indeterminate general conditions which promote the acquisition of virus infections: 'No matter how affluent and civilized, humans were humans and susceptible to viruses that could come from nowhere. In fact, it was easier for a virus to come from nowhere these days' (156). In Shilts's narrative, Africa is thus supplanted by, or made into, 'nowhere' as the place of origin of the virus, as the story moves from seeking the virus's origin to mapping its movements. The underlying position that it was brought into, rather than possibly emanated from, North America is however never called into question. North America thus continues to figure as the victim of the story, the tragic space.

Towards the end of Shilts's narrative, this tragic space is re-figured, as its inhabitants, the gay community, emerge – like the risen Christ – as survivors. The specific form this survivor takes is Cleve, the initiator of the Names Project quilt. Through the resilience, resourcefulness and self-help which he embodies, uninfected Americans are 'won over' outside the frame of a 'political message': 'The quilt also encouraged people to respond compassionately to the plight posed by AIDS, while advancing no overt political message' (619). But there is a message – the message of human suffering, its record. Cleve's message is supposedly simple: 'Americans needed to take care of one another and accept one another, no matter what seemed to separate them' (619). In a quasi-epiphanic ending Shilts asserts, through Cleve, that 'people were coming to understand the value of a gay person's life and the great injustice that had been committed against gay people in the course of the epidemic' (620). Shilts's liberal, humanist position marks the end of his AIDS-in-the-North-American-gay-community narrative in ways characteristic of realist fiction or naturalist drama: an order of sorts is restored, (social) integration is achieved, the crisis is resolved or at least potentially resolvable, politics goes back into the cupboard as a humanist consensus position takes hold:[13] 'The future Cleve envisioned was not so much one of bright triumph, as one of absence of darkness, with the potential of a new dawn ahead, someday' (620).

We live in hope. But some of us more so than others. In an interesting twist to his ending, Shilts separates the AIDS narrative he constructs for the gay community in North America from other narratives as multiple strands and stories emerge. For 'intravenous drug users in the American inner cities' and 'the impoverished masses of the Third World ... riding a later wave of the epidemic, saw the disease as a naturalistic drama with little that could be considered heartening' (620). The notion that the two groups of people identified here – and Shilts jumps from the bourgeois preoccupation with the individual which has dominated his realist account to the 'masses' as he discusses 'drug users' and the 'impoverished masses of the Third World' – view their situation as 'a naturalistic drama' is doubtful. But it serves as a way of separating out the story of AIDS in the gay North American community and other AIDS stories: 'They were separate stories now, the story of AIDS among gays and the story of AIDS elsewhere' (621). The rounding-off of Shilts's narrative reinscribes community specificity and thus difference as a key factor in these stories.

And, in Christ-like fashion, North America and the west are constructed not just as victims and survivors but also as the saviours for the rest of the world, and specifically the 'undeveloped part' thereof. Shilts's narrative comes to a halt in Rakai, Uganda, the final location of his journey. In the beginning lies the end. The image created is of a young man and his child, both suffering from 'slim' or AIDS (here described as a 'wasting disease'). The young man's father is delighted to hear that 'an American journalist knows many of the western doctors working on the disease' (621) for: 'He knows only that the United States is a country of immense wealth, and that the medicine that will save his country and his son will probably come from there. Tears gather in his brown eyes, and he asks, "When will it come? When will there be the cure?"' (621). In Shilts's sentimentalizing narrative North America is first presented as a victim, then as a survivor, and finally as the likely saviour in relation to a disease which supposedly came to the west from Africa, which the west has managed for the most part to contain within one community (gays) and which the west looks set to combat in others, including, ultimately, Africa. Location thus equals more than geographical specificity – it becomes imbued with the meaning of the AIDS narrative at a specific point in time and, beyond that, with the excess of meaning invested in the location which carry the value judgements inherent in the narrative. These decree, for instance, that a certain power relation exists between America and Africa which casts the two continents into particular interdependencies. Secure in his judgements, Shilts generates an epistemic certainty which presents as facts what is at best conjecture.

Through the structural devices Shilts employs and the citational chains involved in these, Shilts anchors his story in narrative conventions which serve simultaneously to assemble and to dissemble. What in the beginning appear to be disjointed fragments, the groundedness of which is guaranteed only through the specificity of the location ascribed to them, soon become a realist narrative in which the map and the journey as well as the naming of specific individuals are the means through which that narrative is visibilized and endowed with a notion of authenticity and truth. The verisimilitude of the identifications of place, time and person supports the truth value of the story – a truth value which reproduces an all-American narrative of overcoming, pulling together, a coming together in crisis but within which, ultimately, individuals and specific communities retain their place within the social hierarchy and networks. The narrative thus reinforces the point made by Peggy Phelan (1993) in *Unmarked* that visibility or visibilization does not necessarily guarantee an acceptance or, indeed, even a recognition of difference but rather that visibilization carries with it the dangers of the recuperation inherent in the citational chains with which all visibilization is inevitably fettered. Shilts feels able to construct an ultimately linear narrative about AIDS. Drawing on a variety of representational conventions which include drama, realist fiction, the detective novel and documentary, he creates the kind of mix associated with what he declares the book to be: 'a work of journalism' (623). This lays claim to a certain truth value while at the same time allowing the kind of dramatization which makes for 'a good read'. Invention and reportage are conjoined to license Shilts's narrative and invest it with the certainty and assuredness which only the use of the indicative, and the proclamation of agency, can legitimate. But such legitimation belies the state of knowledge we are in regarding HIV/AIDS. Its function is not so much to tell the truth as to create a certain narrative effect. Its purpose is to locate and thereby to localize. Shilts's story recreates a journey which never happened. It draws a map or web of connections which has no counterpart in material reality. The connections Shilts makes reinforce particular conventional images of America and of Africa into which the HIV/AIDS narrative is made to fit. Specifying, pinpointing becomes the dominant mode by means of which Shilts seeks to counteract the uncertainties generated by HIV/AIDS.

Strange origins

The forcedness of this narrative constraining is brought out in my third example. On 30 November 1993 *The Guardian* devoted one of its 'Pass notes' to the subject of AIDS. These pass notes, modelled on the idea of providing a series of basic information on a subject so that one might pass an exam on that topic, take the form of questions and answers designed to establish the identity of the subject at hand. The kinds of questions usually asked in *The Guardian*'s 'Pass notes' are a mix of the seemingly objective and the obviously subjective, requiring factual data and opinion in order to create a specific image which is supposedly part truth, part anecdote but in general aims to reinforce the reader's view of what she apparently knows already. The format is thus conservative, intended to provide a thumbnail profile of a known entity. In the instance of HIV/AIDS, however, the pass notes act as a quasi-Foucauldian reverse discourse which trade in uncertainty, parodying their own form. Thus they start with the question of 'age' of AIDS, only to answer it with 'unknown'. The question itself reflects a point of debate among HIV/AIDS specialists who, as part of the process of tracking HIV/AIDS, have sought – unsuccessfully – to establish when HIV/AIDS first appeared.[14] Thus in 1990, for example, *The Guardian* reported that the re-examination of preserved tissue from a man who had died from 'what were then rare conditions' (cytomegalovirus and pneumocystis carinii) in Manchester in 1959 suggested that he had been infected with HIV (Mihill 1990b; Morris 1990). Uncertainty permeated this case since both the identity and the origin of the man who was identified as itinerant through his profession as a sailor (a 'seaman') remained unknown, it was not known how he had contracted the virus, and a 'suggestion that he had been to Africa', implying that he might have contracted the virus there, turned out to be dubious (Morris 1990). The case had been reported in *The Lancet* by three doctors (Corbitt, Bailey and Williams 1990). When the HIV diagnosis asserted by Corbitt *et al.* was subsequently queried in an article in *Nature* (Zhu and Ho 1995), Bailey and Corbitt (1996) wrote a letter to the editor of *The Lancet*, answering the points raised in Zhu and Ho's article and agreeing that 'the strain of the virus in our original extract material is modern' (meaning that it postdated the death of the seaman) and that 'we must conclude that we can find no evidence ... to suggest that the 1959 Manchester patient carried the HIV genome'. Since Zhu and Ho had made the claim that 'clinical material from more than one patient had been referred to them' (Bailey and Corbitt 1996), Corbitt and Bailey's main concern was to refute the suggestion that 'the original published results were in some way synthesised'. Bailey and Corbitt pointed to various laboratory and knowledge constraints they had worked under at the time of their original investigation as explanations for their findings. Their work, as they put it, was 'done in good faith from the outset' (Bailey and Corbitt 1996). This is not in question here. The issue which the case raises, and which the uncertainty articulated in *The Guardian*'s 'Pass notes' regarding the age of AIDS reinforces, is the question of the purpose which pinpointing AIDS's age has and what this implies about constructions of knowledge as they circulate in the western world. Here knowledge of one's age is considered an integral part of one's identity, a way of securing fixity which in itself is constructed as a form of knowledge.

The 'Pass notes' also ask about HIV's origin, answering the question with, 'The Guardian would have a Nobel Prize if we knew the answer'. In other words, a further unknown. Underlying both the questions of age and origin is the notion that the past can illuminate the present and the future, that we know, or at least can understand, the latter two through the former. In his three-part series also in *The Guardian* on 'The Story of AIDS' Mike Bygrave (1993) points to patterns in the histories of infectious diseases to suggest that knowledge of 'the origin of Aids' is important 'not for what it tells us about the past but for what it can tell us about the future'. According to Bygrave, 'Getting an accurate evolutionary perspective on HIV/AIDS has vital implications, ranging from strategies for treatments aimed at the virus mutation, to strategies for prevention' (1993: 32). Explicit in Bygrave's statement is the notion of 'evolution' – the present evolving from the past, and the past thus being usable for making sense of the present – as the underlying principle of knowledge formation. But, as the example of the 'Pass notes' demonstrates, such knowledge formation is implicated in ideological positions which privilege particular visibilizations and readings of the data presented.[15]

In discussing the origin of HIV the 'Pass notes' cite several of the theories posited to explain the emergence of HIV. Among these are that HIV 'originated in US or Soviet laboratories specializing in biological warfare', and infected 'green monkeys' from whom Africans prone to 'the African custom of eating uncooked monkey brain' were supposed to have caught HIV, HIV/AIDS then making its way to the USA 'via Haitians returning home from Zaire'. In other words, Haitians were meant to have caught HIV in Zaire and then infected gay US citizens holidaying in Haiti. Whilst the laboratory hypothesis is instantly dismissed as 'a bit far-fetched' the chain of events leading from African green monkeys to gay American tourists in Haiti is left to stand – possibly because it is also simply deemed too far-fetched to warrant further comment – as the 'Pass notes' move to 'the silliest forecast of the eighties' for which the Royal College of Nursing gets the prize.[16] Ending with a jibe at epidemiological forecastersn the 'Pass notes' state that they would be 'most likely to say ... we have every faith in our mathematical models' and 'least likely to say ... we got it wrong'. The latter is attributed to 'all those research grants up for grabs' which make it impossible to admit failure or ignorance, a reference repeatedly encountered among those questioning so-called AIDS orthodoxies.

A parody of 'potted' knowledge, *The Guardian*'s 'Pass notes' on AIDS of 1993 gesture towards the lack of knowledge which continues to fuel the debates about HIV and AIDS. The overall tone, however, is not so much one of concern as of weariness at the excess of the responses to HIV/AIDS. Most of the 'Pass notes' are taken up with detailing such over-reactions. The first half of the text, for example, focuses on the fear of potential contagion as articulated through the tabloid press who 'went potty', through clergymen who 'turned away people with Aids in fear of divine intervention', 'doctors who refused to carry out post-mortems', the dons at an Oxford college who banned communal drinking from a cup, and police in Scotland who destroyed the car of a man they believed to be infected with HIV. The second half of the 'Pass notes' then centres on the excesses in the theories regarding the origin of AIDS. Both sets of excessive responses, as excesses, point to the distorting impact of the fear of the unknown. Against these distortions are set what seem to be the realities, namely that instead of a million cases of HIV/AIDS in Britain by 1990 there are, in 1993, '8,252 known cases of Aids and 20,590 of HIV'. The question is, what kind of response to this assertion is anticipated? If one assumes that it is 'we got it wrong' – the thing that experts would never say according to the 'Pass notes' – then is that response meant to lead to a more sober assessment of HIV/AIDS? Is it meant to be an antidote to the excesses in response of 'the early years' or is it another form of containment, belittling the HIV/AIDS scare and putting it in its place? The history of HIV/AIDS representation of the 1990s would suggest the latter since the preoccupation with HIV/AIDS which was so dominant in the late 1980s and early 1990s had all but died away in the late 1990s. Containment has become the order of the day.

Containment: knowing its place

The point made by Shilts towards the end of *And the Band ...* that there are now separate stories about HIV/AIDS in different locations has, in a sense, become true[17] as different subtypes of HIV have been identified, and these have been tied to specific locations. Thus Andrew Artenstein *et al.* (1995) reported in *The Lancet*: 'The global HIV-1 epidemic comprises infections from at least nine genetically distinct subtypes of virus (A–H and O), and the distribution of certain subtypes is geographically limited' (1197). S. K. Brodine *et al.* (1995) also asserted: 'Whereas several HIV-1 subtypes co-circulate in many parts of the world, some regions seem to have a predominant subtype. Subtypes A, C, and D are common in Africa, whereas nearly all viruses identified in North America and Europe are B; subtype E predominates in Thailand' (1198). However, the comfort that such specificity might bring through the implications of containment and identifiability is undermined by the fact that Artenstein *et al.*'s article is in fact about the 'multiple introductions of HIV-1 subtype E into the western hemisphere', that is the migration of particular strains of HIV from east to west through, in this instance, military personnel from the Uruguayan Army and Marine Corps sent on peace-keeping duties to Cambodia where, it is concluded, they became infected with subtype E. Three narratives, versions of which are already present in Shilts's (1987) account, are brought together here: infection moving from east to west, the notion of migrancy[18] as central to the dissemination of the virus, and the representation of separate HIV narratives – here, however, in a sense ironically brought together again through the introduction of the originally geographically and demographically contained into new spaces awaiting colonization. Artenstein *et al.*'s conclusions indicate the collapse of the site-specificity implied in the HIV subtype maps drawn above: 'The global dispersion of HIV-1 has been linked to the movement of individuals and populations as a result of natural disasters and man-made conditions (e.g. civil war, tourism, and the drug trade) and the subsequent economic and social changes engendered by these movements … Such movements may lead to dispersion of diverse HIV-1 subtypes into regions previously affected by a more genetically restricted epidemic' (1995: 1198).

One logical consequence of this view is to attempt to restrict human movements, or to control activities of humans on the move.[19] New revelations thus lead to new kinds of surveillance while legitimating old forms of discrimination, and in particular racism. In 1996, for example, it was reported that 'the Israeli blood bank was routinely discarding all but the most rare of blood donations from Ethiopians, because they come from a high-risk HIV region' (Fishman 1996). Fuelled, apparently, by the notion that 'African subtypes [of HIV-1] are already circulating in Europe and there is some concern about the possible spread of the African pattern of AIDS in Western countries' (Galai *et al.* 1997), Ethiopian immigrants became the victims of a new policy of excluding their blood donations since HIV-1 prevalence was judged to be significantly higher in that community than among other Israelis. In a complex article which questions the appropriateness of the policy

Edward H. Kaplan (1998) produces a series of arguments to query the Israeli position, stating, for instance, that 'HIV-1 prevalence in the USA is roughly 25 times higher than that in Israel, yet public-health officials would not consider banning blood donations from US immigrants' (1127). In the main, however, he points to the fact that through the exclusion policy, 'The stigma placed on the Ethiopian community in Israel on account of this policy was substantial' (1128). In fact, it led to demonstrations and riots as the Ethiopian immigrants sought to express their distress at the policy. Following his multi-factor cost-benefit analysis, Kaplan explains that the numbers of infectious donations, that is the benefits, prevented by the routine discarding of Ethiopian immigrants' blood, were negligible (1128) whilst the costs, in particular in human relations, were high. The discrimination exercised through the exclusion of Ethiopian immigrant donors demonstrates the anti-African bias which permeates the countries which perceive themselves to be western. Kaplan, for instance, indicates that although 'virtually all HIV-1 infections among Ethiopian immigrants have occurred among adults who immigrated to Israel since 1991' (1127), recent immigrants constitute just over 41 per cent of Ethiopian Israelis but despite this the whole community is the object of discrimination through the exclusion. In the course of his argument Kaplan moves his terminology from 'Ethiopian immigrants' to 'Ethiopian Israelis'. The latter term suggests a higher degree of integration than the exclusion would indicate. Effectively, what this case demonstrates is the way in which anti-African bias has been allowed to surface as part of an ongoing propagation of the myth that Africa is the source of infectious diseases and specifically of HIV/AIDS.

The western response of containment as indexed in the case of the Ethiopian Israeli blood donors fails to take into account a key phenomenon which contributes to the spread of HIV/AIDS and which is itself very difficult to police: mobility and migrancy. Economic and political factors prevent the hermeneutic sealing of any geographical space. By implication they should therefore also prevent the notion that what occurs in one space has no impact on what happens in another. The need for collaboration across spaces is, however, implicitly and explicitly continuously denied. Culturally, it sometimes seems as if the neat maps of disease patterns continuously produced in medical journals, UNAIDS reports and the like which show clearly delineated geographical regions with national borders conveniently being co-terminous with disease prevalence figures produce a consciousness of divisions that allow a disregard for the realities now faced by the global population regarding HIV/AIDS. In a telling report of the 12th World AIDS Conference which took place in Geneva in July 1998 and which, ironically one might argue, bore the title 'Bridging the gap', Richard Horton describes how 'whenever a speaker from a developing world country rose to talk about an issue ... seats emptied and the hall began to bleed delegates through the aisles and out into the corridors of the conference centre' (122). This appalling disregard for speakers from Africa, India and Thailand[20] and the turning of their backs by western delegates to those viewed as 'other' ignores our implicatedness in the spread of HIV/AIDS. It suggests the continued notion that HIV/AIDS narratives from the west are more important than those from the east or south.

The history of HIV/AIDS to date reveals the desire by the west to read, once again, the map of the world in terms of a social imaginary which makes an imagined 'other' – minimally a French-speaking Canadian, maximally the African continent – the source of an unstoppable contamination. Surface differences, visible and audible differences are made to serve as indexes of other, hidden differences, of which carrying the HIV virus is just one. But the drive towards a linear narrative inherent in this position, the notion that creating maps becomes a way of charting and, indeed, containing (the spread of) HIV/AIDS, has proved impossible. Instead, a multiplicity of parallel stories has emerged which suggests uneven developments regarding the spread of HIV/AIDS on a global level. But these uneven developments are not random.[21] 'The developing world, where 800 million people lack access to health services, bears more than 90% of the global burden of HIV infection' (Horton 1998). Despite the fact that it was in North America and Europe that HIV/AIDS was first identified, it is not those countries which suffer most from HIV/AIDS (Phoolcharoen 1999). The fact that it was in these countries that HIV/AIDS was identified first simply reinforces the notion of the more sophisticated medical machinery which the west has at its disposal, the more effective methods of dealing with the disease. The benefits of these have been extended to 'the developing world' only in very limited ways. In an interesting response to Horton's 12th World AIDS Conference report, Pazè (1998) points out that 'in many places there are not even the facilities to diagnose HIV-1, unless it presents as AIDS' and that since in Uganda, for example, the tuberculosis therapy completion rate is about 25 per cent (1072), 'How can we think that anybody will manage to comply with a complex treatment such as the one recommended for AIDS in places without the most basic facilities?' (1072). In a world where, as Shilts's text would have it, Africa looks to the west to supply treatment solutions, but those solutions are only conceived of in terms of western conditions, 'bridging the gap' appears very unlikely indeed.

The debates about the relationship between HIV and AIDS, Shilts's text and *The Guardian*'s 'Pass Notes' on AIDS indicate a continued attempt to make HIV/AIDS visible and thus to fix it through generating maps which chart the movement of the virus. The specificities of the narratives associated with this visibilization suggest a south to north, east to west movement which is, however, highly contested. The narratives about the history of HIV and AIDS are inadequate in charting the actual occurences of HIV/AIDS. They are themselves site-specific interventions in that they mark points in time and space (e.g. 1987 and North America) when a particular version of the HIV/AIDS story was in circulation. One difficulty is that these narratives are often invested with an epistemic certainty which later 'discoveries' belie. The narratives thus project the temporary and provisional specificity of the visibilization of HIV/AIDS since patterns of movement and infection change. The impossibility of that visibility acting as a guarantor of the fixity and identifiability of HIV/AIDS is reinforced by the mobility of the virus and the non-linearity of its movement. It is therefore impossible to contain the virus through movement restriction. In 1995 Decosas *et al.* pointed out that mobility *per se* was not the issue in containing the spread of HIV but 'the social disruption which characterizes certain types of migration, which determines vulnerability to HIV' (826). In a subsequent letter to *The Lancet* Wolffers and Fernandez (1995) emphasized the importance of 'the paradigmatic shift of viewing migrants as potential carriers of a virus to understanding that migration creates conditions that facilitate HIV infection' (1303). These conditions include dislocation and isolation from traditional environments, the creation of illegal work forces who cannot be dealt with in any 'official' capacity, the creation of all-male environments into which sex workers are introduced, and the construction of dispossessed people with no rights and little access to any form of support.

The question of how to combat HIV and AIDS under these conditions is a difficult one. To the extent that it happens 'elsewhere', that is in other parts of the world than the western one, HIV/AIDS seems to be viewed as someone else's story and one which, however appalling, does not affect 'us'. In 1990, for instance, *The Guardian* carried a report with the headline, 'India losing its battle with Aids' (Fineman 1990). In 1997 *The Lancet* ran a series of reports and articles on 'the global burden of disease' which considered, and sometimes condemned, the World Health Organization's continuing policy of 'making eradication of infectious diseases a priority' (Gwatkin 1997). But, as Gwatkin pointed out, 'Infectious diseases continue to be what matter most for the world's poorest people despite the important progress that has taken place in the past two decades'. These poorest people are found predominantly in the 'developing' world. The desire to eradicate infectious diseases is set against the fact that 'Compared with those in industrialized countries, people in developing countries have little access to treatment for HIV infection' (UK NGO AIDS Consortium 1998). One reason for this, as Michael Adler (1998) indicates, is cost. This combined with the difficulties in treatment management where the taking of '20-30 tablets per day' is required for which both clean water and refrigeration are necessary means that 'Universal access to care and treatment for HIV infection and AIDS is not a reality in the developed world, let alone developing countries' (Adler 1998). In some respects an impasse has developed between 'developing' and 'developed' countries regarding the fight against HIV/AIDS. Calls for interventions are met by counter-claims of the impossibility of such interventions. The stories are different for each country. Thus while President Daniel arap Moi 'scupper[ed] sex-education plans in Kenya' in 1997 (Kigotho 1997) since Catholic bishops and anti-abortionists in Kenya were opposed to sex education, the Philippines 'finally pass[ed] [an] AIDS Act in 1998' (Wallerstein 1998) which provided for a 'comprehensive nation-wide education to break down the taboos surrounding the disease in this staunchly Catholic country'. The idea of a unified strategy to combat HIV/AIDS has long since become a fantasy. This fantasy matches the dream for the finding of – embodied in its search for – a specifiable origin of HIV/AIDS. Simon Watney (1989b) reproduced a point made by the head of Uganda's national AIDS prevention committee: 'There is a snake in the house. Do you just sit and ask where the snake came from? Should we not be more concerned with what action needs to be taken now that the snake is in the house?' (191).

The history of HIV/AIDS to date shows that the past cannot illuminate – and thereby cure – the present since the past does not map neatly on to the present. Even if the sailor who died in Manchester in 1959 had suffered from HIV infection, it is quite unclear what relevance that knowledge could have (had) for the late twentieth century. Retrospective attempts to map the history of HIV/AIDS such as Shilts's *And the Band* ... illuminate the cultural specificities and traditions of the narratives we draw on to understand diseases but in their reproduction of well established cultural myths they defy the kinds of divergent thinking necessary to combat HIV/AIDS effectively. Instead they create the contexts which allow attitudes such as those expressed through Jackie Kay's poetry, discussed in the following chapter, to come to the fore.

Notes

1 Significantly, Shilts attributes this description to a doctor who has spent 'years of battling epidemics in Africa, Asia, and America' (1988: 73).

2 See Patton (1997) for a further debate of this phenomenon.

3 Renée Sabatier (1988) provides one answer, related to the attribution of guilt, in *Blaming Others*.

4 Attacks on pharmaceutical companies and grant-giving bodies are a common aspect of such dissident voices, precisely because of the moneys involved.

5 In 'AIDS and HIV infection in the third world' Treichler (1989) discusses the notion of experiential expertise (64) to suggest the possibility of theoretical sophistication in localized knowledges and to query the efficacy of western medical science as a 'transhistorical, transcultural model of reality' (63) which is adequate to dealing with AIDS in all contexts.

6 Similar debates about the relationship between HIV and AIDS have raged intermittently for many years. In 1990 Nicholas de Jongh commented on one of these in *The Guardian* when a Channel 4 television programme in the UK had 'suggested that the HIV virus did not necessarily lead to AIDS' (1990: 7). In 1993 an extended debate ran between *The Sunday Times* and *The Guardian* when John Illman of *The Guardian* wrote an article in advance of World AIDS Day in which he described *The Sunday Times*'s approach to AIDS as 'akin to believing in medieval alchemy' (Illman 1993a: 2). *The Guardian* then published a list of quotations from what were termed 'AIDS refuseniks' (Torres 1993) and an article by Madeleine Bunting condemnatory of *The Sunday Times*'s 'campaign claiming that the Aids epidemic in Africa, and heterosexual Aids, are both myths, and that the disease does not spread through the HIV virus' (13). Andrew Neil, then editor of *The Sunday Times*, retorted with a letter to the editor of *The Guardian*. The point here is the continued contestation of the relationship between HIV and AIDS which attests to the uncertainty surrounding both.

7 In an article in *The Times* in 1992 Charles Bremner reported on Duesberg stating that he 'speaks with the blithe self-assurance of a dissident who has seen the light, endured banishment for his views and now senses vindication around the corner'. That vindication seems as remote as ever.

8 In 'Influence and power in the media' Tim Radford (1996) discusses people's ability to distinguish 'dangerous rubbish' (1533) from more likely stories despite the fact that 'most of what most people know about AIDS and HIV *is* derived from the media' (1533). He cites the *Sunday Times* articles disputing the connections between HIV and AIDS as an example of media assertions that seem to have no impact on what people actually think ('I do not know anyone who does not connect HIV with AIDS') and suggests that people treat media reports as they treat stories – with a remarkable capacity to 'distinguish the stuff that does matter from the stuff that does not' (1535).

9 Shilts did not himself invent the notion of Africa as the origin of HIV/AIDS. For an account and critique of this notion see Chirimuuta and Chirimuuta (1987) and Miller and Rockwell (1988).

10 John Greyson (1993), the author of the video 'Parma Violets' which was exhibited at the *AIDS: The Artists' Response* exhibition discussed in Chapter 3, created a counter-myth to the notion of Patient Zero in his film *Zero Patience*, a musical spoof on the notion of Patient Zero.

11 See, for instance, Edward W. Said's seminal (1978) *Orientalism* and his subsequent (1993) *Culture and Imperialism*; or Andrew Parker *et al*'s (1992) *Nationalisms and Sexualities*.

12 There have, of course, been a number of cases reported in the press of people deliberately infecting others with the HIV virus, or of at least continuing to have unprotected sex once they had been diagnosed as HIV positive (e.g. Chelala 1992; Mitchell

1992). Kitzinger (1994: 104–6) reports various versions of 'seductive vengeful women' presented in the media. To quote just two examples of the phenomenon: in 1993 *The Guardian* reported that 'HIV "vampires" wreak havoc' – a story about twenty-seven HIV-positive homosexuals and prostitutes in the Brazilian city of Pelotas who were apparently deliberately infecting local residents through sexual intercourse as a way of seeking revenge for their condition. In 1990 *The Guardian* carried several reports (Coles 1990); (Brindle 1990) about an HIV-positive man who had 'abused youths' in London. It was not entirely clear whether the man knew of his HIV-positive status or not at the point of abuse.

13 For an angry denial of this narrative being the most appropriate one see Watney (1997) and Bhatt and Lee (1997).

14 Chirimuuta and Chirimuuta (1987) have extensively, and with specific reference to the hypothesis that AIDS originated in Africa, documented diagnostic problems in relation to HIV/AIDS.

15 A good example of this is the issue of the numbers of high false-positive results from ELISA tests done in African countries where the prevalence of infectious diseases such as malaria and tuberculosis resulted in distorted findings concerning numbers of HIV-infected people (Chirimuuta and Chirimuuta 1987: 53–68).

16 In a letter to the editor, Christine Hancock, the General Secretary of the Royal College of Nursing, subsequently stood by the 1985 prediction cited in the 'Pass notes', stating that 'the comment was made with the best information available at the time and was essential to shock people out of a frightening complacency' (Hancock 1993: 25).

17 One of the foremost medical journals, *The Lancet*, for instance, carries endless reports of site-specific HIV-related stories with headings such as 'HIV prevalence among pregnant women in Kigali, Rwanda' (Leroy *et al.* 1995), 'Finger clubbing and HIV infection in Malawian children' (Graham *et al.* 1997), or 'Philippines finally passes AIDS act' (Wallerstein 1998). These both locate and localize specific HIV- and AIDS-related issues, presenting them as contained, separate stories.

18 In 1995 Decosas *et al.* pointed to the 'keen interest' which had existed in 'mapping the routes of HIV infection' which after 'years of acrimonious debate about where the virus came from' had been abandoned as a 'useless discussion' by the 'health community'. Attempting the xenophobia inherent in this topic, they suggested that 'it is not the origin, or the destination of migration, but the social disruption which characterizes certain types of migration, which determines vulnerability to HIV'. In a subsequent letter to *The Lancet* Wolffers and Fernandez (1995) endorsed this view, stating, 'The paradigmatic shift of viewing migrants as potential carriers of a virus to understanding that migration creates conditions that facilitate HIV infection is very important'.

19 See Decosas *et al.* (1995), Wolffers and Fernandez (1995), and Colvin *et al.* (1995) for a discussion of this.

20 A similar scenario manifested itself in *The Guardian* in 1993 when the first secretary of the Royal Thai Embassy wrote to that paper in response to an article by John Illman (1993b) on HIV/AIDS in Thailand, pointing out that Illman's article neglected 'to mention any of the Thai government's own efforts to stop the spread of HIV' and contained 'stereotypical notions about Thai culture and society'. As Treichler (1989) has rightly suggested, 'Western AIDS discourse transforms a culture so that it ceases to recognize itself but paradoxically becomes recognizable in the West' (42).

21 In 1993, for instance, *The Guardian* ran a story on Haiti in which the reference to 'a rampant Aids epidemic' is just one element which contributes to the representation of Haiti as 'Horror's homeland' where 'Cite Soleil is a hellish place – the Conradian heart of Haiti's darkness' (Tisdall 1993). The reproduction of a mythic image

of debasement is justified through reference to a history in which, so this narrative goes, 'the forcible transplanting of a people far away from their African roots also seems to have deepened the unending Haitian trauma, as with America's own black population. Slavery permanently degraded and disfigured them.' Predictably, there is no suggestion that this applies to the white population of America or the white population of Australia.

5

Alien bodies: HIV/AIDS in Jackie Kay's *The Adoption Papers* and *Off Colour*

... because I didn't fit the description of what they thought someone with HIV should look like, then there was no way that I could have been. (Garfield 1994: 85)

Identity is visibility, a textual production, the condition of both community and annihilation. (Patton 1990: 129)

Knowing the past

As indicated in the previous chapter, Shilts's *And the Band Played On* constitutes an attempt to create a history of the emergence of HIV/AIDS, based on the assumption that that history, as fact, speaks a truth which in turn illuminates the present and foreshadows the future.[1] Knowing the past is thus constructed as a way of understanding the present. A linear relation is established between past and present which replicates the notion of cause and effect, and generates a sense of certainty derived from the supposed predictability of that relationship and the 'progress' from past to present. The fictionality, the imaginary quality of this history-making, is revealed, however, through the representational conventions Shilts employs to create his narrative. These conventions embody certain cultural norms[2] which are in consequence replicated as part of the construction of Shilts's narrative. One such convention is the notion of the unproblematic relationship between past and present.

This notion is troubled in Jackie Kay's (1991) *The Adoption Papers*.[3] Here the relationship between past and present is interrogated through the body which, as in the case of HIV positivity, becomes the site where the interplay of different moments in time is marked as a 'before' and an 'after', but with no necessary linearity between the two. *The Adoption Papers* is divided into two sets of poems, each with their own headings ('The Adoption Papers' and 'Severe Gale 8'). These, on the surface, suggest two separate sections. For reasons I have discussed elsewhere (Griffin 1997) the first set of poems has received considerably more critical attention than the second. However, it is the inter-relationship between the two sets of poems I am interested in here since both sets are concerned with the relationship between past and present and the inscription of that relationship on the body.

The first section focuses on the adoption of a black baby by a white couple, articulated from the three viewpoints of the biological mother, the adoptive mother and the child herself. The second set of poems deals with a variety of issues including lesbian and gay relationships, foreign-ness, the social and economic decline of Britain during the 1980s, parenting, and ageing. It also contains three poems which may be said to deal specifically with HIV/AIDS:[4] 'Dance of the cherry blossom', 'He told us he wanted a black coffin', and 'Lighthouse wall'.[5] Whilst it is possible to consider these three poems in isolation, I think it is precisely their embeddedness in *The Adoption Papers* as a whole which generates their meaning and the contextual framework for this meaning. On their own the three poems capture the mood of the 'dying fall', the melancholic and elegaic quality of an individual death prefigured by a slow dying, in the process of which life is pared down towards that individual and his most immediate relationship/s. I use 'his' advisedly here since all three poems feature a young gay man – representative of the group of people most immediately and sustainedly affected by HIV/AIDS in western countries. Thus 'Dance of the cherry blossom' centres on a gay couple both of whom seem to be HIV-positive though this is never explicitly stated. Both suffer from a disease which is slowly killing them and both know, and joke about, this. The anticipation of death is sublimated by semi-jocular references to 'every couple's dream', the notion that one won't have to wait for the other 'up there' since, presumably, they both expect to die within a short time of each other. The poem foregrounds a sense of the gay couple's daily routines, their companionship, their love-making and their attempts to come to terms with their situation elaborated through trying to find out what happened in the past, who had the illness first, who gave it to whom, squabbling and reconciliation. The image of the gay men as a couple, formally encoded by the use of couplets, is of a settled one-to-one relationship in which both partners are thoroughly focused on each other and 'there's nothing outside' (Kay 1991: 51). The intensity of the entwining of the gay couple may be a function of the disease – it is certainly an antidote to the image of gay men as preferring sex without commitment. However, the concentration on the interiority of their shared lives is also the condition of a life where the present has taken the place of the future. The cherry blossom's dance which acts as the dominant metaphor in this poem figures both as an emblem of the formal device of the couplet and as a mirror of the gay couple's daily engagement with each other. The gaiety of the cherry blossom in spring dancing as it falls simultaneously bespeaks the sense of a premature death and the cheerful moments in the life of the couple as they make love against the background of their impending fate of death.

In 'He told us he wanted a black coffin' (1991: 52) a mother recalls both the last few days of her son's life and his funeral, and earlier periods of his life. The flower motif already present in 'Dance of the cherry blossom' is here repeated in the image of the white lilies on the black coffin, 'Derek's flowers'. They recall the final flower motif in Jarman's *Bue*. The mother, who is represented as understanding of her son's homosexuality as well as of his partner thinks back to her son's infancy and teenage years, trying to remember though 'everything is all messed up'. Again, as in 'Dance of the cherry blossom' where one of the men is trying to work out whom his partner met 'between May 87 and March 89', here the mother is attempting to make sense of the present, her son's illness and death, through the past as she remembers both difficult and joyful instances from his earlier life. Her desire to shield him from physical harm and emotional upset has not been realizable since his life is not hers to live for him. She respects his wishes in life and in death: his request for 'no morphine' as he lies in the hospital trying to savour his remaining days, and his desire for a black coffin. She has always accepted his homosexuality. But her attempts to support him cannot guarantee his life. The mother has to suffer her son's life and death as he has to suffer them – without any obvious sense of cause and effect, without the ability to rationalize those experiences. Comparisons, such as the son's face resembling that of a 'person from Belsen' suggest similarities across situations but these do not explain or justify the events. They simply help to emblematize them.

The son in this poem has the advantage of a supporting mother and a partner. In 'Lighthouse wall' (1991: 53) the persona is alone. His monologue charts his life in the hospice where he moves between consciousness and an awareness of his immediate surroundings, and drifting off into memories of past holidays and the carefree sex he enjoyed prior to becoming ill. His sense of time and his relationship to his body have changed as a consequence of his illness, as they have in the other two poems. All three poems centre on certain kinds of embodied subjectivities, and on the recall or displacement of desire in anticipation of, or following, death. In their focus on specific individuals they might be read as sealed within a particular existence. However, they are also set in the context of *The Adoption Papers* as a whole and as such, as I have suggested above, point to that context as the elucidatory frame for their specific content.

Alien bodies

The Adoption Papers' first set of poems has at its centre an 'alien child', alien because she is 'coloured' in an all-white environment, because she is adopted and therefore not a blood relation, a child of whom one does not know what she will 'turn out to be'. This alien child mirrors, or offers a metaphor for, the alien body or virus which enters the bloodstream of the person who becomes infected with HIV and of which one also does not know what it will turn out to be since AIDS can manifest itself in many different types of opportunistic infections. But unlike the virus which is invisible, this 'alien child' is visible and visibly different – her surface marks her as black. This marking is reinforced through the gash 'down my left cheek' the child receives when she is 'pulled out with forceps' at birth (1991: 10). The violence done to the body in bringing it into the world signals the first violation of its integrity. Thus marked from the beginning, the girl's relationship to her body is problematized through the others with whom she interacts and whose relation to her is determined by the specificities of the differences in their embodiedness. Conceived by a white woman and a black man, the 'natural' white mother gives the baby up for adoption, unable to support her. But since she gives up the child immediately after birth, and indeed leaves her hometown to have her and give her up immediately, it is not the specific child she renounces so much as the embodiment of her relationship with a black man, the visible sign of a sexual relationship outside the bounds of marriage and race. She does not know what the child will 'turn out to be' at the point of decision-making; it is the child's embodiedness *per se* which she has to dissociate herself from. In a related manner, the child's adoptive parents want *a child*, not *this* specific child. They receive a baby when they say, quite by chance it seems, that they 'don't mind the colour'.[6] The specificity of the child's embodiedness, her mark of difference, her skin colour, thus becomes the pivot on which the adoption hinges and which determines her identity. From the adoptive parents' viewpoint, the child's skin colour does not matter since they are desperate for *a baby*, a particular form of embodiedness – for them the colour is irrelevant as their primary desire relates, in a sense, to the size and age of the body they are looking for, not to its surface colour. Ignoring the specific cultural significance of blackness in an all-white, or predominantly white society, they are appalled to discover that the child is 'not even thought of as a baby' – the embodiment of their desire – because she is 'coloured'. Yet in their own lives they also have to negotiate the embodiment of their identity. As communists they feel it encumbant upon themselves to hide the marks of their beliefs (texts by Marx, Engels, Lenin, copies of the *Daily Worker*, a poster of Paul Robeson) when the social worker, embodying one form of institutionalized dominant discourse, comes to inspect their home in advance of the adoption. Still the social worker detects a difference even though the adoptive mother has 'spent all morning trying to look ordinary' (1991: 15). For the baby or the child this is no option. Whilst the adoptive parents can attempt to perform 'ordinariness', the child, who cannot change or hide her colour, cannot perform 'whiteness'. She has to live her visible difference from others, her embodiedness as different from the white norm which surrounds her.[7] In this she has no choice. Her body does not in this respect constitute the body project Brian Turner (1994) for instance refers to, a plastic and malleable entity which one can alter at will.

Reading the body

Some aspects of the body are clearly more alterable, more amenable to interventionary regimes, than others. But in this instance the alteration as it occurs is not related to changing aspects of the body through covering them, or dieting, or surgically intervening, but to negotiating the meanings attached to that body. The child in 'The Adoption Papers' begins to experience herself as an embodied subjectivity through her interactions with others. She experiences the derogation of herself as a consequence of her skin colour from early on. When she is taunted at school for being black, she reacts by defending herself, fighting with the child who calls her names. Aggressivity becomes her means of refusing the attributions levelled at her. It prevents the internalization of the racism she is subjected to. Again and again, as the poem 'Black bottom' makes clear, she has to defend herself against the racism she encounters at school. Significantly, it is the endorsement of that racism from the school, an institutional authority, as embodied in the schoolteacher who automatically assumes the child has done wrong rather than that others have attacked her, for example, which is represented as responsible for how the child is treated. 'The other kids are all right till she starts' (Kay 1991: 25). The taunting stops once the child's adoptive father has spoken to the teacher about what is going on. Racism, the poem makes clear, is not innate but learnt behaviour, fostered through its endorsement by authority figures and institutions. Like the adoption agencies which take as their primary focus the skin colour of the infant, making judgements of her (un)desirability *as a baby* on the basis of that colour, so the teacher makes judgements of the child on the basis of her skin colour. In both instances the judgements are the same: negative. The child's appearance becomes the source of how she is constructed. The body is thus *made* alien through being singled out in ways which draw attention to the specificities of that body, and which embue those specificities with particular meanings. These meanings are not random but systematic and mutually reinforcing, arising from cultural formations which precede the body.[8] When the child is not given a part in *The Prime of Miss Jean Brodie* it is implied that this is because black people cannot play white people (the reverse has, of course, been practised for centuries). Such appropriations trouble the cultural prescriptions which demand separation and the continuous enactment of visible difference as difference along hierarchized lines. Analogously the child, being black, is expected to be a good dancer and asked, like a minstrel, to contribute to the school show. The teacher, exasperated by the child's inability to get the steps right, 'shouts from the bottom / of the class / Come on, show/us what you can do I thought / you people had it in your blood' (1991: 25). The teacher's racist prejudices lead the child to interrogate her subjectivity, her embodiedness: 'What Is In My Blood?' But, as the cover of *The Adoption Papers* makes clear, knowing what is in your blood does not necessarily elucidate its meaning since that meaning exceeds its physiological constraints. The front cover of the volume – its image coloured on black – shows chromosomes, normally invisible to the human eye[9] but here made visible through techniques of amplification, colouring and fixing. This visibility of the chromosomes, of 'what is in the blood', tells the viewer nothing of the chromosomes' specific genetic meaning, for instance. Being able to say what is in the blood therefore has no immediate explanatory power[10] – it simply defers the interpretive moment that will give meaning to what has been visibilized. The instability of meaning which attaches to the image of the chromosomes thus replicates the instability of identity generated in the child through the teacher's remarks.

In interrogating her subjectivity, the child has to negotiate her adoptive parents' position which is to deny the importance of her skin colour, the racist attacks of which she is object at school and which make her skin colour overridingly important, and her sense of self within an all-white environment.[11] In the face of the coercive force of the socio-discursive regimes which the school exposes her to and which decree that 'in a few years time you'll be a juvenile delinquent' (1991: 25) and the sublimatory screening from that regime which her adoptive mother engages in, the child has to arrive at a position which will stabilize her sense of self *vis-à-vis* these discordant discourses. One immediate difficulty is that in the child's environment there is nobody who looks like her and with whom she might therefore physically identify. This is akin to the experience of many gay and lesbian teenagers who feel themselves to be 'the only one' in their environment. 'The only female person' she has seen who looks like her is Angela Davis: 'Her skin is the same too you know' (1991: 27). For the child Davis represents an ideal; being 'as brave as her' becomes something she aspires to. Like the child, Davis is in an adverse situation – imprisoned for her beliefs, she is on 'America's Ten Most Wanted People's List'. The ambiguity of the phrase 'being wanted' with its implications of both desire and horror reflects the ambivalence with which the child, too, is met in her environment, desired by the adoptive parents, rejected by racists at school. But in the child's life Davis herself *is* 'just' an image, not part of the everyday reality which surrounds the child. Since that everyday reality does not include other black people, the child experiences a dissociation from her embodied self which is relived when she looks in the mirror. She expects the mirror to show her what she sees every day. But the 'mirror' everyday life holds up to her is 'white' – the self she sees in an actual mirror is black. The disjunction this experience creates generates a momentary destabilization as the child gives herself 'a bit of a shock' and, looking in the mirror, says to herself, '*Do you really look like this?* / as if I'm somebody else' (1991: 27).[12] That sense of alienation from the embodied self is reinforced through the absence of others like herself, or even knowledge about them, in the child's environment. Angela Davis, it turns out, is unknown to the other children – 'Who's she?' they ask. The child's identification with the unknown does not allow for the triangulation of identifying with someone recognized by others which reinforces one's sense of the integrity and stability of self. The child is thus constructed as perpetually at odds with her environment, finding resemblances, which the real does not yield, only in the symbolic.[13]

What is in the blood?

In 'The Adoption Papers' the body's surface is one source of alienation. Looking different becomes a means of being defined as different. But it is not just the meaning of the surface of the child's body which is in question; what is underneath, too, is the object of public interrogation. When the teacher proclaims, 'I thought / you people had it in your blood', she repeats the notion of an embodied subjectivity in which the outward sign, the skin colour, is supposed to attest to an inward disposition which repeats itself in others outward signs such as the ability to dance. A structured judgement thus emerges, akin to the Möbius strip invoked by Elizabeth Grosz (1994) as an explanatory model to describe embodied subjectivities: 'The Möbius strip has the advantage of showing the inflection of mind into body and body into mind, the ways in which, through a kind of twisting or inversion, one side becomes another. This model also provides a way of … rethinking the relations between the inside and the outside of the subject … by showing … the torsion of the one into the other, the passage, vector, or uncontrollable drift of the inside into the outside and the outside into the inside' (xii). The teacher conflates outside and inside, reading the one into the other and back again, in a process which is indicative of the way in which, as Grosz puts it, bodies are open to 'cultural completion' (xi). Completion, however, suggests the making of a whole, the finishing of something, a process of integration, potentially something positive. But the establishment of the child's subjectivity is not merely a matter of adding on and completing but also of resistance and modification, development and change as a function of resistance to that which is imposed or attributed from the outside such as the racist remarks of the teacher. The phrase 'cultural completion' thus does not fully express the process of interaction between inside and outside which makes that embodied subjectivity. 'Cultural intervention' or 'extension' might therefore be a more appropriate phrase.

The child's body is variously read by the different people whom she comes into contact with. But she is not just a passive recipient of those readings. The readings she is exposed to such as those of her skin colour expressed by her adoptive mother and by the teacher and other children respectively, which offer divergent positions on the same material reality, promote an active disposition on her part to explore her self. Self-objectification, looking for points of identification as a way of understanding one's identity, or rather the attribution of identity to which the child is object, becomes her way of dealing with the social ordering the child experiences. She decides that she wants 'to know my blood', to understand what is 'in her blood'. She wants to understand how her external corporeality relates to her interior physicality. Whilst that desire is couched entirely in physical terms, concerned with 'what diseases / come down my line' (Kay 1991: 29), with 'the mother's nose and father's eyes' (Kay 1991: 29), what is visible on the outside as a function of the inside, it articulates a desire for 'social completion' (Grosz 1994: xi) since, without that completion, 'the old blood questions about family runnings' (Kay 1991: 29) have to be answered by the adopted girl with 'I have no nose or mouth or eyes / to match, no spitting image'. Instead, the girl experiences herself as sealed off from the social reciprocity guaranteed through the blood relations: 'my face watches itself in the glass' (1991: 29). The girl has no 'other' of similar appearance to complete herself through; the fantasy of social completion remains just that,[14] a desire which is not actualized. The girl's desire for knowing what is in her blood is not fulfilled. She makes an effort to trace her biological mother but they never meet. Since the mother is white and not mixed-race like the child, meeting the biological mother would not, at the level of surface appearance or skin, produce the 'spitting image' the girl is looking for. The impossibility of being completed by an other is reinforced through the doubling of the girl's parents (biological and adoptive, the same but not quite the same) effected through the adoption. In asking in whose image she is made the girl is offered the choice of the biological parents as explanatory of her genetic make-up, and her adoptive parents as keys to her psychical disposition. The Möbius-strip-like interrelationship between the physical and the psychical precludes either set of parents as the only necessary other to complete the self. The multiplication of others who might be like oneself thus forestalls any closure to the desire for completion. There is no synonymity, only approximation.

The uncertainty of history

The desire for social completion emerges in 'The Adoption Papers' as a desire to know the past, to have a history that will explain the present. A similar desire for completion, for knowing one's past or one's history as passed down through one's blood, characterizes the relationship between the two gay men in 'Dance of the cherry blossom' (1991: 50–1). Here what is 'passed on' is the HIV virus, and the question is both about how the persona's partner became infected (the persona does not suggest that he might have become infected first but admits that his partner 'thinks I gave it to him'), and who of the couple 'had it first'. The presentation of the routines of daily life suggests the dailiness of the questions asked about the 'origin' of the illness. As with the adopted child there is no resolution, just the iterativity of the questions, recognised as futile ('I know I'm wasting precious time / But ...') but asked none the less, again and again.

Both 'The Adoption Papers' and 'Dance of the cherry blossom' share an assumption that one's history is inscribed on and in one's body, but that that history is not necessarily knowable and, that ultimately that history will not, as a matter of course, illuminate the present. For, the question one might ask is, why do you want to know who had it first or who your biological parent is?[15] What would such knowledge do? The knowledge of the past demanded by institutions such as the medical establishment or registration offices produces specific forms of epistemic and ontological certainty, suggests a fixity which both the fact of adoption and HIV/AIDS belie. The past influences the present but it is not a guarantor of that present – it does not seal its meaning. Knowing who gave it to whom does not alter the fact that both of them are getting worse. But the possibility of an attribution of responsibility to an 'other' deflects from the self and the notion that embodied subjectivities arise out of dialectical contexts in which self and other impact on one other. The desire for knowledge of the past then is about the positioning of the self in relation to an other. The alien body, whether as a visibly different, adopted child, or as an invisible virus circulating in the blood, seems to demand a (re)reading of the social to accommodate that body. Part of that (re)reading is the quest for origins.

Naturalizing the 'alien' body

The impact of the social on the corporeal, its Möbius-strip-like quality of an outside-in, inside-out movement, raises questions about the relationship between nature and nurture, between what is innate and what is acculturated.[16] *The Adoption Papers* utilizes the analogy between the alien, or alienated, body of the adopted child and the circulation of the virus in the body as it simultaneously articulates the naturalization of certain social phenomena within dominant discourse and denaturalizes these through a complex process of significatory reversals and inversions.[17] In so doing Kay engages with the debates about 'the family'[18] and specifically maternity which occupied, and continues to occupy, much of 1990s public thinking.[19] Asking 'what is natural', Kay's poems indicate that, since the body is open to social completion or extension or intervention, it is *produced* rather than *is*, and the question should therefore be what is natural*ized* rather than what is 'natural'. What is naturalized, constructed as 'natural' is, for instance, the desire for motherhood – hence the devastation of the adoptive mother when she discovers that she cannot do 'that incredible natural thing that women do' (1991: 10), that is conceive a child by means of heterosexual intercourse. But the articulation of that desire may happen only within very specific socially sanctioned boundaries, also made natural through a whole variety of legal, medical and other discourses. Not to be able to have a child through heterosexual intercourse thus becomes a 'secret failure' about which there is something 'scandalous' (1991: 10). However, the implied significance of the biological bond as, *inter alia*, a guarantor of mother love is queried not only through the fact that adoption is an option but also through the representation of the adoptive mother as loving. Though people may say 'it's not like having your own child though is it' (1991: 23) for the adoptive mother, 'there is no mother and daughter more similar ... closer than blood. / Thicker than water' (1991: 34).

Marking the body

The adoption agencies as public bodies who maintain certain social norms enforce a particular idea of the ideal family[20] made explicit in Kay's poem through the couple seeking to adopt being repeatedly rejected as not suitable. According to their criteria, the couple fails to fulfil the 'norms' (1991: 14) such as being churchgoers or having a specific level of income which are constitutive of the 'ideal family'. When the adoption eventually occurs, there is nothing 'natural' in terms of naturalized-because-socially-sanctioned about it. The adoption is effected through and despite a subversion of all the naturalizing conventions intended to protect 'the family'. The white couple whose political persuasions and secularism place them outside the 'ideal family' adopt a black baby, making manifest their difference from those around them and foregrounding their family as produced, as made up or constructed rather than 'natural'. Moreover, *The Adoption Papers* indicates that there are many ways in which one can become a mother: through adoption, through artificial insemination or, indeed, through baby-snatching. None of these is a 'natural' way of acquiring a child but all are the result of the 'natural' desire for motherhood. Bodies thus, as Grosz puts it, 'always extend the framework which attempts to contain them, to seep beyond their domains of control' (1994: xi). In so doing they become marked bodies, bodies singled out for their non-compliance with the imaginary norm.

The marking may take physical forms, or be realized through other sign systems such as the use of derogatory language. Through this marking individuals acquire a sense of self which they need to negotiate as part of the process of integrating the various, and potentially contradictory, discourses of which they are objects, into some sort of provisionally stable identity which includes a sense of bodily integrity. In Kay's poetry the marking of embodied subjectivities is always a source of suffering. It is also always aligned with the individual's experience of his or her body. There is no marking that does not entail violence or a violation. In the three poems which portray gay men dying from AIDS,[21] their bodies are marked both by their history of sex and by their present condition of sickness. Their current physical suffering is linked to past bodily experience, sometimes ironically so, as when one of the couple in 'Dance of the cherry blossom' is attributed the line, 'I'm dying for fuck's sake' (Kay 1991: 50). In each poem an attempt is made to make sense of the present through reviewing the past. In 'He told us he wanted a black coffin' the mother's reminiscences about her son are first of a body always being marked and injured (an abcess; falling of a wall; being called 'a poof'), and then move to memories of the well, joyous body of her son which becomes conflated with 'the man in the hospital bed ... his face a person from Belsen' (1991: 52). That conflation of various states of being, the afflicted younger self, the healthy, younger self and the sick older self suggest a continuity which is the continuity of the mother's reminiscences as much as a continuity of a specific personhood. In its deliberate selectivity it is also an index of the role of the imaginary in the formation and maintenance of that identity. The memories which the mother conjures up do not explain what happened to her son – they mark points in time but not causal connections. Similarly, the persona in 'Lighthouse wall' explores in his mind his past and the present in hospital. Bodily sensations from the past such as feeling cold swimming in the freezing Atlantic sea translate into feeling cold through being sick but the continuities established here are refracted through different bodily states, the healthy one and the sick one, in which these sensations acquire different meanings. Kay seems to signal that at the level of meaning it is all in the mind but what is in the mind are states of the body. These are not amenable to monolithic interpretations since they cannot be contained through narratives of cause and effect as Shilts would have it in *And the Band Played On*. The past can therefore act neither as authenticator nor as guarantor of the present. 'Past' and 'present' encapsulate different moments whose relation is indeterminate. The present body does not necessarily provide clues either to the past or to the present. The black child's skin colour does not reveal what colour her father or her mother were, nor does it show her adoptive parents' colour. What it marks is a visible difference from all those around the child who are not black. That difference becomes a means of affirming the norm as the differenced person is made to feel excluded through being derided. The teacher's comment about the ability to dance supposedly being in the black person's blood establishes a particular relation between the visible body and that which is invisible, what is 'in the blood'. Here inside and outside are meant to affirm each other. The girl's inability to dance queries the attribution of particular physical competences as race-specific, simultaneously making the girl potentially different both from white and different from black people. This double alienation requires a negotiation of the physical and the cultural within the social which makes the child subject as well as object of her own gaze in the effort to understand her particular embodiment and subjectivity. Subjection to the teacher's view condemns the girl to self-alienation; resistance to that view results in dissociation from the authority which the teacher embodies and the need to establish a sense of self separate from the projections of the teacher.

The existence of the body marked as different generates violence, violence from those who view themselves as invaded by an alien presence, and counter-violence, both physical and non-physical, from those thus attacked. The maintenance of an idea of a norm, so Kay's poetry suggests, cannot operate without violence and violation. But there is no safety, either outside of or within that normative discursivity. In Kay's poetry the mother, emblem of a certain embodied normativity, is always ultimately unable to protect the child. This is not so much an indictment of the mother as a recognition of difference and of female subjection in western culture. Nowhere is that clearer than in Kay's poem 'Dressing up'. Here Kay constructs a symmetry between a cross-dressing son and his mother who is the object of domestic violence, which simultaneously suggests and belies any similarity between them. Both mother and son dress up for a Christmas dinner, the mother in a sober navy dress, the son in black stockings and a bright red feather boa. Both mother and son are victimized, the mother for being a woman, the son for cross-dressing. It is their appearance, their embodiment, which is met with the violence that permeates the household. The mother's victimization is inscribed on her body through her black eye, a memento of the physical violence to which she is subjected by the father. The son's inscription of difference on his body takes the form of drag – it is his way of putting space between himself and his parents, creating a difference.

Unlike the mother from 'He told us ...' this mother is unable to cope with her son's enactment of difference. The symmetry of their victimization does not lead to an identification of mother with son. Instead, the mother 'others' her son by commenting on his appearance with 'You look a bloody mess you do' (1991: 57). The irony of that comment, reserved for the reader as the twist in the tale, seemingly escapes her but the fact that she has a black eye invites the reader to consider who precisely is in a mess here. It also points to the fact that the idea of the norm is itself not a guarantor of the integrity of the body or its inviolability. There is ample room for violations which are socially sanctioned and function to reinforce boundaries and hierarchies of differentiation within those normative structures, chief amongst which is 'the family'. Difference as disciplined and punished is allowed the space necessary to affirm normative behaviour, and to demonstrate the incorporation of that norm in the figure of the mother through her abjection of an other, the cross-dressing son.

Kay's poems probe intimate relations, 'the family' and partnerships. Within these the body marked by AIDS is differentiated out from a wider social context. The focus on the individual, his immediate environment and experience seals that person off from others as he advances towards death or, as in the case of 'He told us ...', has already died. That isolation is the enactment of a bodily separation from the social. Interaction with others affirms a corporeal future which the disease puts in question, as the future recedes and the relationship between past and present is interrogated. When in 'Dance of the cherry blossom' one partner tells the other that in heaven he will have him every night, the desirability of the unknown future which is heaven is reinforced by reference to the body, the having of 'your glorious legs / your string hard belly, your kissable cheeks' (1991: 51). The material reality of that body, however, is already in question, the shoulders caving in and the breathing being trapped as the man cries, suggesting a body 'getting worse', the changing of the body as part of the illness. The image of the two men making love and rolling on the floor 'like whirlwind' projects both a sense of energy and of lightness, the weight loss associated with AIDS. Memories of the past and fantasies about the future are set against the present. In 'He told us ...' and in 'Lighthouse wall', too, a bodily present – if not presence – is set against a bodily past. The persona's sense of self is articulated through bodily experience. In the drifting mind of the man in 'Lighthouse wall' the past becomes the present. Associatively, he slips between diverse states of mind (awakeness and dozing) and different states of imaginary and actual embodiment. The differentiation between actual and imaginary world gives way as friends 'start to merge together'. The remembered body becomes the ill man's means of remembering himself. The remembered body is not a body in isolation however but an interacting body, a body involved in articulating and enacting physical desire, a desire consigned to the realm of the imagination since the man can no longer act on it. Much as he would love to pinch the nurse's bottom, for instance, he cannot do so. The image the man conjures up of the past is of a fit, sexually active body. In his debilitated state he is 'so aware / of my body shrinking'. His present body bears only an imaginary relation to his past one, since it bears no resemblance to that past body now conjured up only through his daydreaming. The past as imagined or remembered by the man has thus become interiorized – memory has no visible traces. It acts as an invisible bulwark against loss, precluding its finality.

Figuring loss[22]

In *The Adoption Papers* Kay's poems on adoption and on HIV/AIDS centre on the psychic and physical negotiation of an inevitable, either already effected or impending loss which cannot be avoided. In the three poems dealing with HIV/AIDS, this loss has a different meaning from that in 'The Adoption Papers' since the former are concerned with a decline unto death while such death does not figure in 'The Adoption Papers'. Here loss (for instance of the biological mother's loss of the child, or the adopted child's loss of the natural mother) and the possibility of moving on from such loss are enacted through ritualized burial and fantasies or dreams of reunion. In the poems concerned with HIV/AIDS, different conditions prevail. In 'Dance of the cherry blossom' the persona mourns the foreshadowed death of both himself and his partner through obsessively going over the past in order to pinpoint the occasion of infection and blame. Mourning emerges here as an iterative process; in the shadow of death, where overcoming is not an option and reconciliation with the idea of death implies resignation. The iterativity of the process keeps the lost object which is not actually lost yet but whose loss is impending in place and present.[25] Part of the difficulty of the daily negotiations between the two gay men is the simultaneity of the continued existence of the beloved object and the expectation of its loss. This simultaneity occasions both affection and aggression, leading to alternate interactions of arguments and lovemaking. They are copiously enacted in the sealed-off existence which the two dying gay men lead. This interiorization of their existence matches 'the loss of the social world, the substitution of psychic parts and antagonisms for external relations among social actors' which Butler (1997: 179) describes as an effect of melancholia and which explains the representation of the mourning subject in Kay's poetry.

In 'He told us he wanted a black coffin' it is the mother who is mourning her dead son. Here the lost object, the son, is kept alive through and in the mother's reminiscences. Part of what the mother mourns is her inability to keep her son from harm, to maintain his integrity as a body and as an embodied subjectivity. That inability, not so much due to a lack of will but because of its impossibility, is the story of her and of his life. Attacks on her son, his negative experiences, become her impoverishment, the embodiment of the impossibility to shield him. That impossibility affirms their separateness as subjects. It enables the mother's mourning to be tempered by her recognition that she cannot incorporate her son into herself or take his place. She could no more 'take the abscess out / of his five year old mouth and put it into [hers]' (Kay 1991: 52) than prevent his becoming infected with HIV. His separateness from her is thus repeatedly brought home to her, affirming the split between the self and other which supports difference. That recognition does not, however, lead to abandonment but to support, even in the face of an otherness unto death. The mother's experience of the *impossibility* of protecting her son becomes the basis for her ability to cope with his death. In remembering the son's laughter and asking, 'who'll laugh now?' (1991: 52) the mother envisages the present as future – a future without her son. Similarly the question about the song 'he sang at the school concert / (what was it?)' (1991: 52), which indicates her forgetting, points to an internalization of the lost object and his incorporation into a psychic landscape with more and less significant landmarks, an accommodation of that which is lost within an interior landscape that identifies the past as past. This is not the equivalent of abandonment or disavowal but rather the acceptance of suffering since no compensatory measures are possible. 'It doesn't seem that long ago', the final words of the poem, ambiguously reference both the son's death and his past life when he sang at the school concert. The contraction of time into a single point signalled by this ambiguity is effected by the son's death which interrupts time as a chronological unfolding through the establishment of stasis, an unvarying state of being dead. This stasis re-orders the past from sequentiality into simultaneity, with the mother's reminiscences repeating through remembering the impossibility of the preservation of her son's psychic and physical integrity as an iterative process that structured their relationship. His death is thus an affirmation of the specific structure of their relationship.[24] Her fulfilment of his wishes after death represent the continuation of that structure of separateness and supportiveness.

In 'Lighthouse wall' the persona mourns a former existence as a healthy sexualized and sexualizing body whose identity was confirmed through the sociality of sexual encounters. The persona's sense of his declining body generates a sense of doom which is intermittently alleviated by the memories of his past (self). Utilizing the present continuous tense, Kay constructs the persona as enacting his past, acting it out in his reminiscences which offer an antidote to his present state. The recall of the past becomes the persona's way of preserving the lost object, his sexually active, healthy former self, which, when experienced as loss during the more conscious periods, leads to depression and a sense of pointlessness. The inability to perform, the objectification of the self through the hospitalization process, the condemnation of the self to a passivity which renders the physical as a process of necessities regulated from outside rather than by an agentic self, changes the persona's relation to time. His inability to control his situation beyond the encounters encoded in medical discourse as 'normal' within a hospital or hospice setting means that he cannot determine the rhythms of his life any longer. As a result time starts to expand and contract seemingly randomly. The goal orientation of the persona's earlier life has given way to an enforced aimlessness, conditioned by his bodily state and his having to abandon control over his life. As in 'He told us he wanted a black coffin', the absence of a future makes the past the only way in which the lost object having existed can be confirmed. And as in 'He told us ...' past and present are collapsed as the persona drifts into inhabiting his former self, made present in the process of reminiscing. The will to live is stronger than the resignation inherent in accepting one's impending death. The persona, observing his weight loss and reduction in body size, imagines that he 'might just disappear / into the white cotton' (1991: 53), merge with the hospital bed and become an undifferentiated nothing. The fear of this leads him to 'hold onto the hands of friends' but they also lose their individuality as his perceptions weaken. His body is failing him. But his mind continues to conjure up the past self with whom he becomes synonymous again in the process of remembering.

Virus in rebellion

In Kay's HIV/AIDS poems, mourning represents a way of coming to terms with death. By the time Kay's most recent collection of poems, *Off Colour* (1998), was published, her engagement with 'the virus' – about which there are four poems in this volume – had taken a very different turn. *Off Colour* plays on tropes of racism and illness as comparable states of bodies constructed as at odds with their environment, the same combination which informed the poems of *The Adoption Papers*. The collection starts with a mock-hypochondriacal poem, 'Where it hurts', which figures the body as a 'bloody battlefield', the pathologized body who is 'sick to death of being sick' and who is in rebellion against the regimes and rituals which occasion and regiment the body's sickness. This body, far from submissively accommodating its conditions, rages against them, mocking a culture which constructs the body as perpetually unwell. Its exuberant aggressivity, presented as a tirade which simultaneously invites the addressee to engage with its sicknesses and articulates its fed-up-ness at being ill, becomes a celebration of life in the face of death, here transfigured into the desire for 'a fucking great fucking big death' (Kay 1998: 12). The poem's excessiveness in its totalizing claims, part of the parodic language which attacks a culture where the body has become a constant source of worry,[25] signals the expenditure of grief, the refusal to internalize and incorporate sickness into the self and thus to succumb to it. The body's resilience despite having been 'sick since time immemorial / since the days of the plague' (1998: 9) raises questions about the nature of illness, its own historicity and its cultural conditioning. The poem articulates the rituals, verbal and non-verbal, which accompany, possibly constitute, the body marked as ill, the repetitive question about how one is, for instance, or the ritual of treatment. These rituals establish the body's illness as performative, here understood as the iterative enactment of processes associated with being sick. The ritualization and acculturation of illness contains it in specific forms but this does not change the underlying situation, namely that of the perception of the body as sick.

In 'Where it hurts' that sick body is not the specific, individualized body of the earlier poems but a body abstracted across time, the body as a phenomenon in culture and history. The body is thus the subject of the poem, both as topic and as persona. The recognition of the way in which that body, despite its continuous illnesses, has resisted death so that death becomes a spectacular fantasy rather than a lived actuality is expressive of the fighting spirit which the body manifests. Defying all illnesses, the body has prevailed – it continues to live against all the odds. This is a body of hope, not of death. This body does not revile itself. Rather, it parades its conditions only to defy them, to live through and beyond them. It not so much refuses as reviews its losses, revelling in the extremes of experience which signal a culture at odds with its bodies. The excess of that experience where people try 'everything' to regulate the body, where nothing is what it seems ('what's a smile but an attempt to hide tears') and where everything can be turned into a cliché, is a mark of the over-investment in the body which characterizes our culture. The anticipation of illness, the expectation of loss, so the poem suggests, acts as an antidote to a life 'away from the worry – the body' (1998: 10), a life in which the potentially or actually sick body is not at the centre of our preoccupations. The continuity of that preoccupation, in the context of successive waves of illnesses ('My illnesses just keep coming; going out-in, in-out'), is also the mark of its overcoming since it defies the expectation of the sick body as sick unto death. This is a body sick through life, permanently assaulted but never defeated. As such it raises questions about the role of the imaginary in the pathologization of the body. The body, produced in culture, exhibits that history.

The effect of this representation of the body is to move Kay's poetry from the melancholic and elegiac contemplation of loss as discussed in relation to the previous HIV/AIDS poems to a position in which the need to re-vision the experience of the body becomes the implicit demand. The encoding of that experience is socially determined. Social determinancy becomes the source of meaning in *Off Colour*, 'the condition of community' as Patton (1990) puts it. Kay does not address HIV/AIDS directly in *Off Colour*, but her poems 'Plague' and 'Virus' (there are four of the latter) invite consideration of HIV/AIDS since the words 'plague' and 'virus' have now become so powerfully associated with HIV/AIDS. 'Plague' goes back to the times of the actual plague, describing the reaction of a plague victim to having her door marked with a white X, signalling an infected household. Despite the fact that most neighbours' doors are marked just like the persona's, the persona's desire is to be done with the plague, to have the mark removed or painted over, to be no longer marked. This is not unlike the body's desire in 'Where it hurts' to get away from attributions of sickness. But the poem suggests that it is impossible to move from a marked to an unmarked state: not only is the white cross likely to remain visible even after it has been painted over; the very arrangement of the bones in the grave, the crossing of the arms on a dead body mean that the mark of the plague remains inscribed on the body even in death through the ritual of how the body is buried. The body thus manipulated from the outside cannot escape its marking. This inescapability is reiterated in 'Virus *' where the addressee is invited to 'say the words / come first' (Kay 1998: 24). Illness is constructed as 'the alphabet' which dictates that the end, being a corpse, is the inevitable result of 'being got' by some disease, with the disease that will get you already known before you are born. The marking your body experiences, the illnesses it may die of, are identified like letters in the alphabet, existent prior to your existence and seemingly independent of any embodied subject[26] who is invited to 'say you were targeted by a particular / virus' (1998: 24). The invitation to say it, to produce the words which predate the experience, is intended to point to a prior scene, relieving the individual of blame or responsibility for his or her condition. But if you have to say it, that might suggest that this situation is not as self-evident as it might seem, that there might be another way of looking which suggests that you have created the conditions of your demise. Pre-empting that accusation is a way of absolving yourself. It does not answer the question of origin, though, since the poem suggests that you might 'say it was was written / ****in the stars****' (1998: 24). There is, then, no explanation other than that of prior existence which can be offered for the condition we are in, for the disease that kills us.

The second 'Virus **' poem, focusing on leprosy, juxtaposes thinking about the experience of leprosy now that leprosy no longer occurs in Europe[27] with the reality of leprosy as lived in the past. As in 'Virus *', the focus is on language: 'the word shakes you up. / leper' (1998: 36). The lived reality of the leper colony has, as a phenomenon of the past, become nothing more than a phrase suggestive of 'fiction', something which is not real. Leprosy has receded into the mind, 'a terrible imagination', something that exists only as words though once it bespoke the actual embodiment of a physical condition. Implicit in this poem may be the notion that illnesses come and go – their terrible reality turning into mere words as they become contained and are eradicated. The poem thus gestures towards a future when the embodiment of a particular condition, be it leprosy or HIV/AIDS, is no longer a lived reality but a (newly) imaginary entity, existing only in language. Effectively, this poem considers the relationship between language and embodied condition from the other end of the continuum envisaged in 'Virus *'. Where in that poem language precedes the condition, here language is all that is left after the condition has been obliterated.

By 'Virus ***' (1998: 45) it is no longer those affected by disease who speak but the virus itself. The virus in question appears to be that of the bubonic plague: 'Bubo! It's all go.' Its accent suggests a local specificity – Scotland – which is reminiscent of the geographical boundaries drawn around the appearance of HIV/AIDS in diverse locations. But that specificity is intercut with an indiscriminate attitude towards potential hosts: 'ma host the rat snuffs it, / A kin a ways switch tack.' Man, woman or child, 'it's awrasame tae me'. Here it is the virus's habits rather than people's disposition or behaviour which determines its movements, and the rate of these movements is predicated upon the speed with which those infected succumb. The virus as devious and triumphalist destroyer ('Wey ma canny disguise / A make sure human hosts / drap like flies') notes the social relations which specify bodies ('Somebody's dochter. Somebody's Maw.') but it is their corporeality, their 'sweet blood bodies', that are its delight. Without empathy, the virus's view of humans is tied to its impulse to survive.

It is the human perspective on what the poem details which refracts that position into one of judgement.

'Virus ****' is more enigmatic, creating three scenes in which relations of time, space and body are obscured through a pared-down use of language, involving in stanzas one and three repetition with variation. The first tercet identifies a space, 'love nest', qualified by changing possessive pronouns, 'our', 'your' and 'their', which – contrary to the idea that such pronouns identify ownership – in fact obscure that ownership. For whose love nest is it? Following the grammatical pattern of first, second and third person plurals, the pronouns move from most to least intimate. The sequentiality of grammar and language is not matched by a sense of successive inhabitants of the 'love nest' which may or may not be a single space. Indeterminacy rules. The poem immediately preceding this one, actually entitled 'Love Nest' (Kay 1998: 53), suggests co-habitation of people and pests, and the dismay of people at successive invasions by different kinds of pests. The second stanza of 'Virus ****', consisting of just two lines, parades a list of sexually transmitted diseases, a scene of infectivity. The third stanza contains a love scene in which the variants are time and pronouns. Two bodies are implied through the bellies which are kissed but it is 'my belly' first, 'her belly' next, and 'my belly' last. It is unclear who does the kissing or what the sequence signifies – is it a virus, or a sexually transmitted disease, or the lover, who 'kisses' these bellies[28] – are they giving it to each other, to use a phrase from 'Dance of the cherry blossom'? And: what is the significance of the time sequence – does it signify the end of an affair, already potentially indicated through the changing ownership of the love nest, or is it concerned with the process of infection, arising out of mutuality and corporeal intimacy?

The specificities of *The Adoption Papers* as presenting an image of melancholic contemplation of young gay men and their partners and relations facing death from AIDS have given way in *Off Colour* to a much less elegaic, and in some respects unsentimental, engagement with the body, driven, perhaps, by the changes in knowledge about HIV/AIDS we have witnessed between the early 1990s and the late 1990s. *The Adoption Papers* defies the binarisms between the alien or other and some 'natural' self or social structure through highlighting the naturalization which bodies undergo, a procedure emblematized by the adoption papers themselves which constitute a verbal construct regimented through particular categories that are intended to 'naturalize' a formal procedure. In the process Kay uncovers the violence and violations implicit in the enforcement of normative ideas. The resistance to incorporation which these normativities demand are signalled through the impossibility of changing the marked into an unmarked body without changing dominant discourse itself. This is evident in Larry Kramer's theatre work which, as I shall discuss in the next chapter, utilizes conventions of theatrical representation that both subvert and confirm the power of what Butler (1993) describes as 'the forcible citation of a norm' (232).

Notes

1 For a critique of this view of history see Hayden White (1973; 1978).

2 See, for example, Barthes (1986a; 1977) and Young (1981) for structural analyses of texts which expose the conventions and cultural norms inherent in narrative.

3 Jackie Kay is a black lesbian writer who has written plays, poetry, books for children and a novel, *Trumpet* (London, Picador, 1998). She lives in Manchester with her partner, the poet Carol Ann Duffy.

4 HIV/AIDS is never named in Kay's poems – their presence an inference the reader is invited to draw. It may be that Kay is trying to avoid the labelling or stereotyping which naming engenders, or to suggest that the label is inadequate to conveying the experience.

5 'Lighthouse wall' references Lighthouse, a centre for people affected by HIV and AIDS, which officially opened in London in 1988 (Cantacuzino 1993).

6 This contradicts the adoptive mother's assertion to the child, intended to be reassuring, that the child was *chosen*. In fact, it was allocated as an undesirable object to parents who did not fit the normative criteria of the 'ideal family'.

7 See DuCille (1996) for a discussion of black women's experience of the relationship between skin colour and identity.

8 Ahmed (1998) discusses the specific meanings which attach to 'coloured' skin.

9 Gillian Beer (1996) analyses the change in the status of the eye as an increasingly uncertain instrument of perception in the context of developments in nineteenth-century science. This, in turn, raised questions about the relationship between that which is visible and that which is not, between the outside and the inside. See also Nast and Kobayashi (1996).

10 The human genome project constitutes one attempt to defy the epistemic uncertainty arising from our inability to map DNA fully, to know what is in the blood.

11 Valerie Mason-John (1991) quotes Kay as saying, 'most black children brought up in a white environment will experience some form of psychological distress. It's hard to get a strong sense of being black and proud when there is nothing to reinforce this notion' (38).

12 In a subsequent poem, 'Somebody else' (Kay 1998: 27), the topic of self-alienation, the experience of being simultaneously self and other, is revisited.

13 The meaning of the symbolic as the site for finding resemblances is explored in relation to gays and lesbians in Sedgwick (1990).

14 Several of the poems in 'The Adoption Papers' relate to the fantasy of meeting the biological mother.

15 The cultural imperatives behind this desire are indexed in an article by Meg Henderson (1990) in which she describes her experiences of adopting.

16 Grosz (1994) of course queries this binarization, suggesting an interrelationship which goes beyond the demarcations signalled here. Utilizing that dualism is simply a way of making the argument clearer, not of subscribing to those boundaries.

17 A key stylistic device Kay uses to accomplish this is nature imagery which often takes

the form of analogies (as in 'Dance of the cherry blossom'), metaphors and similes In contexts which are considered 'unnatural' within dominant heterosexist discourse, for instance, such imagery naturalizes what seems unnatural to some. By imbuing other instances such as people's hostile, racist reactions to the mixed-race couple also with natural images Kay's work points to the complexities of what is naturalized and raises questions about the idea of what is natural.

18 One version of 'The Adoption Papers', published in 1991 in a book on lesbian photography (Boffin and Fraser 1991), explicitly queried ideas about the conventional family through its place of publication, a book aimed at lesbians by lesbians, alone.

19 These debates have taken many forms. For some of these, published in the year preceding the publication of *The Adoption Papers*, see Frost and Watt (1990), Jacques (1990) and Grove (1990).

20 See Sherman (1990), Mihill (1990a) and Aldridge (1990) for a discussion of the issue of transracial adoption which featured prominently in the British press in the early part of 1990.

21 Kay produced these poems at a time when AIDS was still seen as a syndrome affecting predominantly gay men in western culture, and where the inevitable consequence of becoming infected with HIV was considered to be death – 'dying from' rather than 'living with' being the operant phrase then.

22 This discussion is informed by Butler (1997), especially chapters 5 and 6.

23 See Butler (1997) for an elaboration of the function of mourning in the formation of the self.

24 For an apposite discussion of the representation of women in general and 'mothers' in particular see Kitzinger 1994.

25 That troubling of the body, especially the female body, is recorded in the emergence of an expansive feminist literature on the subject which includes among many others Bronfen (1992), Butler (1993), Duncan (1996), Grosz (1994), Grosz and Probyn (1995), Martin (1987), Shildrick (1997), Birke (1999), Price and Shildrick (1999).

26 This replicates the relation between subject and object, or author and text, as articulated in Barthes's (1986a) 'The death of the author', which reverses the conventional notion of the author as arbiter of meaning through pointing to the prior existence of language.

27 The last leprosy hospital in Europe (in Bergen, Norway) was closed in 1946.

28 Within a lesbian aesthetic 'the belly' as emblematic of female sexuality is associated with Gertrude Stein's extended poem *Lifting Belly* (rpt Tallahassee, Naiad Press, 1989).

6

In-direction: the new agit-prop of Larry Kramer's theatre

Disease does more than rob the body of function: it also chips away at identity ... The image in the mirror is no longer familiar. (Valdiserri 1994: 9)

There is always something missing in the meeting with the other who is necessary to the constitution of the self. (Tyler 1997: 249)

When asked how he would like to be remembered Larry Kramer replied: 'As a man who fought as hard as he could to make the world a better place for gay men and lesbians and people with AIDS' (Greenstreet 1995: 46). Kramer is indeed a combatant in the fight against HIV/AIDS and this fight, as his *Reports from the Holocaust* (1994) makes clear, has cost him dearly, both personally and politically. His style of fighting is in-your-face, assertive, aggressive, offensive (as opposed to defensive) – he is not known for his indirection. Differences about this, especially with Paul Popham, one of his fellow activists at Gay Men's Health Crisis (GMHC), led to his break with that organization which he had helped to found in 1982 with five other gay men (1994: 22). As Kramer describes it: '[Paul] knew he was right and I knew I was right. He was a much better team player than I'll ever be. I'd been a film producer. I thought I was producing GMHC. He'd been an army officer. Both of us were accustomed to getting results and, in very different fashions, having our own way' (1994: 32). This description points both to Kramer's interest in spectacle, here referenced as film production, and to the issues of sameness and difference which inform all of his work and writings, including that for the theatre. Popham and he are similar yet different – their differences finally forced them apart.

Kramer wrote *The Normal Heart* (first performed in 1985) in the wake of his departure from GMHC. In *Reports* Kramer quotes a friend of his as maintaining that he, i.e. Kramer, 'was subconsciously preparing this break – that [he] wanted to write what was eventually to become [his] play *The Normal Heart,* and that this was the only way [he] could allow [him]self to do so without feeling guilty' (1994: 59). This suggests a degree of deliberation, even if subconscious, which Kramer's plays, both *The Normal Heart* and *The Destiny of Me* (first performed in 1992), would to some extent belie because of the way in which within them he revisits the ground he has (in the case of *The Normal Heart* in particular) just left behind. However, as Carole-Anne Tyler (1997) points out: 'repetition … is not about the return of (or to) the same, but the recurring encounter with a traumatic lack of identity and similarity, the enigma of desire which is the result of our difference from others and even our self' (259). It is this enigma of desire within the wider context of staging HIV/AIDS that I wish to explore in relation to Kramer's plays since, as I shall argue, it is this which informs Kramer's activism and theatre, and determines both the direction and the indirection of his plays.

Having experienced a traumatic lack of similarity between Popham and himself, Kramer revisits his then recent experiences of expulsion from GMHC in his plays. This recurring encounter, with the iterative experience of trauma, is however mediated through its theatricalization. It is given a different form and it is re-shaped, both through re-telling the events related to Kramer's involvement with GMHC in a new medium, as theatre, and through re-framing that narrative in terms of a parallel one, that of the central character Ned's relationship with his brother Ben.

Re-staging the self

Kramer's break with GMHC meant that he had, as he himself describes it, 'lost [his] official soapbox' (1994: 59), his platform for his political activism.[1] In searching for a new location, the theatre appeared to offer an alternative way of specularizing his views, of writing 'something about my experiences since the epidemic began' (1994: 65). With a sense of being 'placed on the front line of history in the making' which resulted in feelings both of obligation and desire, Kramer wanted to produce something which would be 'out in the world as quickly as possible' (1994: 66). Hence the play. Effectively, this move enabled Kramer to relocate his activism into another space and to resignify the meaning of his experiences in GMHC through bringing into focus another story which functions both as a mirror and as an opposite to his relationships within GMHC – the story of his relationship with his family, in *The Normal Heart* centred mainly on his relationship with his brother, in *The Destiny of Me* extended to encompass his brother, father and mother. Having been cast out and thus 'invisibilized' through the process of expulsion from GMHC, Kramer was seeking, again but differently, to make a mark, to re-visibilize himself and regain control in a situation where he had lost it. One difference, this time, was that the product to be created, a play rather than an organization, required a subject position of Kramer which was not the same as that of being a founding member of an organization in which he would be actively involved. The play offered both a less totalizing and a more totalizing position: less totalizing because once written it might be produced by others[2] and performed in places separate from Kramer; more totalizing in that the play would be his word. Kramer's plays became a means for re-staging the self, and specifically his self, within the context of his personal history and the wider socio-political history of AIDS activism.

Sander Gilman (1988a) suggests that the fear of collapse and sense of dissolution which informs western images of disease can be countered by the subject through 'project[ing] this fear onto the world in order to localize it and, indeed, to domesticate it' (1). Gilman maintains that through this externalization 'the other', the construct, takes on the potential of dissolution. Among the 'structures we employ to exorcise the fear that we may lose control' are 'the rigid forms of art' (2). Art as 'an icon of our control of the flux of reality' (2) acts as a bulwark against the dissolution that threatens through disease. I would suggest that in Kramer's case art, in this instance theatre, acted also as a means of refiguring the self at a point of crisis.

Issues of control

When Kramer founded GMHC, he wanted to take control of a situation, the increasing threat of HIV/AIDS to gay men, about which he thought not enough other people, whether the state and the medical professions or gay men themselves, were doing anything. In the face of a lack of focus and direction or goal-orientation, making visible through organizing was a way of trying to control,[3] of dealing with the sense that 'the wounded, diseased subject of modern knowledge seems unable to cure or take care of himself' (Braidotti 1991: 132). But such visibilization brought with it also externalization and objectification, a splitting of the created object, GMHC, from the subject, Kramer, which rendered that object no longer the same (as the subject), i.e. synonymous with the subject, but different and separate from him. As an organization, especially once tax-exempt,[4] GMHC had to conform with regulations which contradicted Kramer's perceptions of what the organization should do and be. Split from himself through the founding act, GMHC was not the same as Kramer any longer but different from him. The object of external regulation, as well as the structure through which a range of people attempted to combat HIV/AIDS, GMHC could no longer be controlled by Kramer in accordance with his views of how campaigning around HIV/AIDS should proceed. Following Kramer's break with GMHC, the creation of *The Normal Heart* may be thought of as the antidote to what happened with GMHC, as Kramer's attempt to reassert control through creating something new (the play) but also through creating something in his image, for, after all, the play is an externalization of or from self. Having gone through one process of creation which meant splitting and the painful recognition of difference, Kramer, in writing the play, went through that process again. His objective remained, in a sense, the same: to raise consciousness about HIV/AIDS and thus activate people into seeking to combat the disease. But the medium through which he was now seeking to propagate his message, the 'means to message', had changed. The theatre became the new domain in which Kramer sought to locate his activism.

Kramer's new agit-prop

In turning to the theatre as the means of promoting HIV/AIDS consciousness Kramer engaged with a visualizing practice which, to use Cindy Patton's words, 'administer[s] categories already in place through another discourse' (1997: 193). Theatre as a visualizing practice comes complete with a range of discourses, categories and frameworks which constitute the history of that medium. These structure the meanings of its productions and reference histories of representation which create an internal dialogue between the past and present of performance. They also determine its performativity, that is the simultaneously iterative and transient specificity of performance. This is evident in some of the critical writings on AIDS drama which have emerged during the late 1980s and early 1990s such as John Clum (1992) or George Newtown (1989). Clum's focus on the parallel between *La Dame aux Camélias* and AIDS dramas serves, in his words, to 'demonstrate[ ] how realistic drama has, from its beginnings in the mid-nineteenth century, placed sexually active characters within the realm of disease as well as that of the normative discourse of sexual morality' (48). Clum maintains that through this process 'The body of the AIDS patient, then, becomes a principal player in a moral allegory as primal as *Everyman*' (41). The historical precedent is thickened by references to a version of *Hamlet* which featured a 'Person with AIDS' (40). Similarly, Newtown in his article draws on Greek tragedy as well as Goethe's *Faust* to analyse the ways in which the relationship between sex, life and death has been presented in different dramatic genres, specifically comedy and tragedy. Such an imbrication of AIDS drama in the established discourses of theatre entails both opportunities for, and limits to, the possibilities of interrogating the regimes which govern theatrical representation. Yet, one might argue, a theatre working for social change needs just such possibilities of interrogation.

The locus of the performance, the theatre itself, sets potentially limiting, particular parameters for such an interrogation since it presents a spatially bounded field and attracts, depending on venue and production, particular audiences. This has consequences for the kind of performance and effects which can be produced out of Kramer's plays.[5] Cindy Patton (1995) analyses the differential construction of self (disease-free) and other (diseased) in the discourses of tropical medicine and epidemiology. Her reading of these discourses provides an interesting analytical frame for the interpretation of the use of theatrical space and discourses as a means of rendering HIV/AIDS visible. Patton contends that both tropical medicine and epidemiology are concerned with mapping and thus visibilizing disease through correlating spaces with populations. The same, in spacio-social terms, might be said of the theatre, where, conventionally, different spaces, i.e. the auditorium and the stage, are designated for different groups of people, the audience and the actors. In her essay Patton starts from the position that 'there has been ... an overemphasis on the actant-subject and a relative lack of consideration of the stage or context or field of the performance' (181). She distinguishes between tropical medicine and epidemiology on the grounds that 'compared to epidemiology, tropical medicine, as a performance on an already secured terrain, is less labile, less subject to intervention by resistant forces' (183). Epidemiology, according to Patton, is performative since it is 'an actant within a place in which the constitution and reproduction of citational chains is constitutive of power' (183). Where tropical diseases are located on the terrain of the other, in colonized spaces, over there, epidemics can occur anywhere: 'Bereft of a stable *place* of pathology, epidemiology must constantly construct and correlate populations and subpopulations in order to make epidemics visible' (187). While tropical medicine correlates a distanced colonized space with disease and the other from whom one has to remain separate to bound disease, epidemiology lacks such a place and therefore constructs imagined communities as a means of collapsing body and space so as to make the epidemic visible and potentially containable. However, 'Disease may radiate out from a place – an epicenter – but it is not proper to it. An epicenter is unstable and uncontained by definition' (187).

The theatre as a space both maintains and threatens to collapse the distinctions Patton makes between tropical medicine as performance and epidemiology as performative and thus constitutes a potent, if deeply problematic, location in which to play out AIDS dramas. On the one hand, the stage in conventional theatres represents a bounded, already secured and stable terrain; plays, on the other hand, are performative in that they move from stage to stage, secured in part by the citational chain which constitutes the history of theatre, its productions, and its canon of plays. To the extent that plays are performative, on the move, they, like the epicentre of an epidemic, are the centre which radiates out and occupies diverse (theatre) spaces. The capacity for each new locale or stage to become a new centre (Patton 1995: 186) radiating out to 'yet more periphery', and the conflation between body and disease in a given – if unstable – space, makes the theatre a particularly conflictual terrain as stability in the form of space, history and canon collides with the instability of the performative text, the production and the audience.

The effects of this collision[6] are forcefully demonstrated in Robert Bradley's (1992) account of the incidents surrounding the production of *The Normal Heart* at Southwest Missouri State University in Springfield in November 1989.[7] The play was chosen for performance because 'not enough had been done on campus and in the Springfield community to make the public aware of AIDS' (362). Thus designed as an intervention, it attracted the wrath of the Vice-President of Academic Affairs and the State Representative Jean Dixon who demanded that the performances should be cancelled or the play be censored as prescribed by her. Things escalated from there, resulting in rallies and counter-rallies, sold-out performances and, in a particularly appalling act of violence, in the burning down of the house of one of the student organizers of an on-campus group who supported the production of *The Normal Heart*. The homophobic arguments against the production focused extensively on issues of ownership: 'Do you want your tax dollars to promote homosexual, anti-family life-style? Why would these state employees and officials approve using your tax money to promote homosexual political agenda in our university?' (Bradley 1992: 363). One might argue that the university and its theatre as a bounded space were here constructed as colonized stable terrain, in line with the discourse of tropical medicine. In this context, certain audiences expect to see themselves, mirror-like, reflected in the productions rather than as some opposite which they do not wish to recognize as anything than 'other'.[8] Since audiences themselves are to some extent unstable entities, only certain audiences in the end – those who attended – saw themselves reflected in the play; those who voiced their opposition relegated the contents of the play to the status of other. The arrival of a particular play therefore put the assumed stability of the terrain of the theatre in question and for some members of the Springfield community raised the issue of how to police the boundaries between an assumed heterosexual, disease-free self[9] and an assumed homosexual, diseased other.

The attacks on individuals associated with the production surfaced two important issues. Firstly, because the play was produced in a bounded space in a conventional production manner, it was identifiable with a particular group of people – the actors, producers and supporters of the play. This rendered them visible and attackable. Otherness thus became concentrated in them and made them the objects of vilification.[10] Secondly, the attacks on individuals associated with the production and its defence highlighted the conflation between body, text and space as well as the fear, illustrated as mentioned above in the burning down of a student's home within the community of Springfield, that what the otherness of the play represented might be a spill-over of a threatening other into the 'taxpaying' community which or who might contaminate it. In that respect the production was treated like an epidemic the location of which had shifted, threatening the boundaries imagined by the 'taxpaying' community and thus, ultimately, constituting a possibly unexpectedly, particularly effective intervention, since, as Bradley details it, 'The campus and community awareness level and desire for information about AIDS [has] never been higher. The director of the university health clinic said that in the four weeks before the production the clinic had given out more information on AIDS than in the entire [previous] year' (369).

Theatricalizing HIV/AIDS

One of the ironies of this experience was that *The Normal Heart* was accused of presenting 'an anti-family life-style' (Bradley 1992: 363). Nothing could, in a sense, be further from the truth. Whilst this rhetoric serves to maintain an imaginary boundary between the homosexual 'them' and the heterosexual 'us', it rests on a complete level of ignorance of what *The Normal Heart* asserts in relation to 'the family'. For, as I shall argue below, it is precisely that assertion, to be discussed more fully shortly, which creates part of the problematic of and a certain indirection in Kramer's new agit-prop. However, in order to make sense of this problematic it is necessary to understand the theatre traditions on which Kramer draws first and I turn to these now.

In April 1987 Kramer gave a speech as part of 'Epidemic, center stage: a forum on the role of theater in AIDS' in which he took on the mantle of 'message queen' to describe his engagement with theatre. Personalizing his position, he maintained:

> I don't think it's the playwright's or the novelist's or the filmmaker's responsibility to deal in ideas or rhetoric or political meaningfulness ... No, I hold no Marxist views about the creative responsibility, even though I might seem to live by them. I only know that at this stage of my own life, with death so palpable and continuously close, I only have time ... to be − a message queen. (1994: 146)

In his speech Kramer simultaneously disavows the notion that *all* artists have a responsibility to engage with matters that have 'relevance to the lives we lead' (147) and asserts 'we just might survive if only each of you could become a message queen too' (148). As in his plays so in this speech Kramer is driven by a recognition of difference (not everybody produces politically relevant work) coupled with a desire for sameness (everybody *should* produce politically relevant work). Kramer's reference to a 'Maxist view of creative responsibility' is important here as it points to a tradition of political theatre within which Kramer's work might be placed, that of agit-prop or agitation and propaganda.

In fact, Kramer's plays, in the main realistic in style, articulate *two* traditions of theatre,[11] both with their own and, in terms of each other, contradictory discourses and imperatives: agit-prop and naturalistic theatre. Agit-prop is a part of the tradition of political theatre, a form of theatre intended to lead to social change through the incitement of the viewers to understand, and hence have the basis for changes in, their situation. Sometimes by, and usually for, those who are disenfranchised or (economically) disadvantaged in society, agit-prop was a theatre form of the left pioneered by Erwin Piscator in pre-1930s Germany. Ewan MacColl describes it as 'giving a new meaning to the term "non-violent direct action"' (Goorney and MacColl 1986: viii).[12] In Kramer's case the desire for direct action goes hand in hand with a powerful fighting spirit which is expressed through the vehemence with which he articulates his convictions and the means, 'borrowed' from the traditions of agit-prop, which he utilizes to project the reality of HIV/AIDS.

Chief among these, in *The Normal Heart*, is the use of the walls in the New York production of that play, to present facts about AIDS, a measure akin to the wall newspapers *inter alia* associated with the dissemination of certain kinds of information in China during the Cultural Revolution but also a visualizing practice commonly used in the political theatre of the first half of the twentieth century. Indeed, Piscator (1929) begins his work *Das Politische Theater* (*Political Theatre*[13]) with the following lines:

Von der Kunst zur Politik
Meine Zeitrechnung beginnt am 4. August 1914.
Von da ab stieg das Barometer:
13 Millionen Tote
11 Millionen Krüppel
50 Millionen Soldaten, die marschierten
 6 Milliarden Geschosse
50 Milliarden Kubikmeter Gas
Was ist da 'persönliche Entwicklung'? Niemand entwickelt sich da 'persönlich'. Da entwickelt etwas anderes ihn. (25)

[From Art to Politics
My time scale begins on 4 August 1914.
From that point onwards the barometer kept rising:
13 million dead
11 million cripples
50 million soldiers on the march
6 billion guns
50 billion square meters of gas
What is 'personal development' in this context? Nobody 'personally' develops there, all by himself. Something else/other develops him.([14])]

Exactly as Kramer is to do more than fifty years later, Piscator begins with figures, figures the magnitude of which, their sheer volume, force him, as they do Kramer, to re-cast his existence in the service of the need for change. Piscator, like Kramer later, is swept up by the events around him. His numbers mirror Kramer's numbers, both as a device, and as a sign of the genocide, in Kramer's case of people with HIV/AIDS, and of the Holocaust to which Kramer refers throughout his writings and which align his work with the period, the First and Second World War, about which Piscator writes. However, whereas Piscator moves from art into politics as a consequence of the context in which he finds himself, Kramer is driven by politics, or his exile from a particular kind of politics, into theatre as the cultural practice which will enable him to produce a reproducible message about the apathy with which the AIDS crisis is met by politicians and populace alike.

This apathy, it should be noted, is not a matter of indifference, but, as Thomas Yingling (1991) puts it, 'AIDS shares more, finally, with genocide than with plague ... [since] the benign neglect of government agencies makes the epidemic a passive-aggressive act on the part of rational society' (306).

The writing on the wall so to speak, which features in *The Normal Heart*, points to the size of the problem which Kramer seeks to address. Similar numbers-related points are made within this play and in *The Destiny of Me*, as various characters like Emma, the doctor in *The Normal Heart*, or Nurse Hanniman in *The Destiny of Me*, detail the numbers of dead and sick, the amounts of money spent by the US government on health-related matters, and other quantifiable issues. Yingling (1991) describes this phenomenon as 'the mathematical sublime' (292). However, the overall effect of these numbers, in part literally as a result of their spatial positioning, in part through the parallel narratives[15] which Kramer's plays invoke, is to function as a *backdrop* to the action which takes place on stage and which, in contradistinction to the ascending numbers of those infected with HIV and those dying from AIDS, focuses on the dwindling numbers of survivors and their impending deaths. As Gregory Gross (1992) puts it: 'The descending numbers do not serve to flood the audience's consciousness over the size of the plague. Instead, the declining size of numbers, moving from the big to the small, draws a funnel-like bead on the individual character' (65).[16] The contrary motion between ascending and descending numbers thus neatly encapsulates a rhetorical strategy used by Kramer both in his speeches and in his plays of juxtaposing the impersonal in the form of figures and facts related to quantity with accounts of individual experiences. It also generates the contradiction which determines the impact of Kramer's plays. For whilst the numbers appearing on the walls reference agit-prop, the focus on the individual points to the naturalistic bourgeois theatre which places the heterosexually invested, conservative and conserving family at the centre of its concerns and evacuates all those who differ. Thus a significant function of naturalistic bourgeois theatre is to establish sameness and difference, and to police the borders between the two, ultimately preserving the status quo. In this respect it is diametrically opposed to the aspirations for social change inherent in agit-prop.

Conventionally, the final expulsion or splitting off of the different from that which epitomizes the bourgois family represents the resolution of naturalistic drama's central conflicts. In *The Normal Heart* these conflicts appear in two guises: as the issue of differences among the activists of GMHC and in Ned's family, specifically in relation to his brother. In *The Destiny of Me* these conflicts are dramatized both in terms of Ned's fights with government institutions (the symbolic parental figures)[17] and in the replay of the dynamics in his family. The scenes which establish difference and splitting in relation to GMHC are painfully presented, or re-played,[18] in *The Normal Heart*, especially in scenes eleven and thirteen where the differences in strategic thinking between the character Ned Weeks (Kramer's on-stage persona) and Bruce Niles (Kramer's play version of Popham) are argued through. Weeks insists that a confrontational style is more effective than acquiescence and compliance. Bruce refuses this line, suggesting that Ned has 'no scruples whatsoever', is '"merchandising" the epidemic', makes an impossible association between the Holocaust and the HIV/AIDS epidemic, and is anti-sex (1987: 2/13, 65). Ned counters this line of argument by pointing out that being gay is about more than sex and that gays needs to organize systematically in order to achieve visibility and thence recognition.

The different positions taken by Ned and Bruce are presented as a product of their very different life circumstances. Ned is an 'out' gay man whose income is derived from various sources of self-employment and careful investment (by the end of the second play, *The Destiny of Me*, he is unproblematically described as rich) while Bruce is closeted and a corporate man. Ned is fully aware of the impact this has on the difference in their strategic thinking but he is unable to accept closetedness[19] and all its implications as a position.[20] He is constructed as passionately wanting others to be the same as himself, fighters, and as finding it difficult for others to be different from him in this respect:

> BRUCE. You don't have any respect for anyone who doesn't think like you, do you?
>
> NED.   Bruce, I don't agree with you about this. I think it's imperative that we all grow up now and come out of the closet. (1987: 1/5, 24)

Coming out of the closet, or being outed, is a situation Bruce fears because at Citibank where he works his 'boss doesn't know and he hates gays' (1987: 1/5, 27). According to Tyler (1997) the notion of 'outing' someone or coming out, intimately bound up with the activities of ACT UP, the organization Kramer helped found some time after he had left GMHC, is associated with an assumption of an essential identity, revealed through the act of 'outing', which asserts that those who are outed should desire what we desire, should be the same as ourselves. But, as Tyler suggests, such a position ignores the fact that 'The same does not repeat itself without a trace of difference that unsettles the identity of the subject hailed by a name or image (mis)-recognized as the self'

(243). Since our sense of self depends on a recognition of ourselves *as* ourselves and of ourselves as ourselves *by* others, the subject both in relation to self and in relation to other is always already split. This means that the desire for, or assumption of, sameness between self and other, as evidenced in Kramer's work, is – in Tyler's words – 'a fantasy': 'The community of signifying clones[21] whose identities are clear, communications transparent, and desires identical is therefore a fantasy based on the repression of differences within both the self and the community' (1997: 249). This does not detract from the fact that organizing as a community on the basis of certain shared characteristics is politically necessary and efficacious. However, in *The Normal Heart* Ned is constructed as desiring sameness and as able to recognize difference but, within certain parameters, as unable to tolerate it. The consequence is that he becomes alienated from those around him. Effectively a clash of desires is generated between Bruce and those like him who want to operate in one way, and Ned who wants to proceed differently. This provokes crises since the need for the other to validate the self is undermined by being rejected by the other, the experience Ned has to cope with when evacuated from GMHC. Through paralleling Ned's experiences in GMHC with his family history, specifically in *The Normal Heart* with the history of his relationship with his straight brother, Kramer produces an explanatory commentary on Ned's behaviour within GMHC, which locates that behaviour in his family background and the familial dynamics of the bourgois family. This reinforces the notion that 'beyond and before the self is the founding other' (Tyler 1997: 234), a founding other here constructed as the bourgeois, heterosexually invested family.

Family relations

In a conversation with his lover Felix, Ned replies to the latter's question, 'What happens when people can't be as strong as you want them to be?', 'Felix, weakness terrifies me. It scares the shit out of me. My father was weak and I'm afraid I'll be like him. His life didn't stand for anything and then it was over. So I fight. Constantly. And if I can do it, I can't understand why everybody else can't do it, too … Okay?' (1987: 2/7, 36) In this exchange three key points are made by Ned, namely that he

- is afraid of weakness
- aligns weakness with his father and is afraid of being or becoming like him
- is afraid of not amounting to anything, like his father.

Ned's life is marked by a fear of the sins of the father being visited on the child.[22] His father Richard failed, from Ned's viewpoint, to represent paternal authority and was undistinguished. In *The Destiny of Me* this failure is explained by Richard's story of his relationship with his own father. On his deathbed[23] Richard tells Ned that '[he] never had a father either' (1987: 3, 66). Richard's father turned almost literally into the castrating father figure when as a mohel, with Richard acting as his assistant, he made a mistake during a circumcision which haunted him and Richard for the rest of their lives. This mistake effectively eclipsed Richard's father's patriarchal legitimacy since it undercut both his authority as a mohel and his status as an accountable male in the Jewish community and in his family: it prompted him to run away. In making Richard 'memorize all the Orthodox laws', of which Richard significantly cites only those relating to masturbation and to same-sex relationships,[24] and through his running away, Richard's father disrupted the homosocial bond between him and Richard to such an extent that Richard, who in the light of all of this is revealed as a potentially gay man, could cope only by adopting a position of self-loathing and pronounced homophobia. Richard is thus constructed as a victim of a certain cyclicity whereby his own father's sins were visited upon him and he in turn victimized his son Ned.

The origins of Ned's need for others to be like him and his inability to tolerate difference is thus located in his relationship with his father Richard in which Richard is characterized as inadequate, and Ned as afraid of turning out to be like the father, a failure in a certain kind of self-accepting masculinity. Ned's assertion of difference from the father operates on a literal-biological as well as a metaphorical basis. In the latter context it is the state in all its institutional manifestations which proves to be weak – unwilling to fight HIV/AIDS because it, in terms of its closeted officials, cannot accept homosexuality as legitimate. Driven by a reaction against 'the father', Ned seeks refuge among biological and symbolic 'brothers'. *The Normal Heart* is thus also a play about fraternity and the need to establish relations of equality with biological and symbolic brothers in a context where the father, as both symbol and 'real' person, is absent, indifferent or dead but continues to fuel the action, including the interactions between the brothers.

Most of *The Normal Heart* is given over to the exploration of Ned's relationships within GMHC. But the play's ending, as discussed below, with the affirmation of the enduring nature of Ned's relationship with his straight blood brother Ben, already prefigures the shifts of emphasis which occur in *The Destiny of Me*. By *The Destiny of Me* the focus is much more, as its introduction states, on '"family" slash "memory"'

(1993: xi). In consequence the relative weighting of the agit-prop versus the naturalistic theatre elements changes from *The Normal Heart* to *The Destiny of Me*. In the introduction to the latter play Kramer states that he began the arrangements for the production of the play when he thought he was dying, a move not unlike Jarman's making of *Blue*. As the title of *Destiny* indicates there is a shift in terms of a move towards a much more hermeneutic, closed structure. *The Destiny of Me* sends the viewer or reader both backwards and forwards on a circular track which is 'me'. In the beginning lies the end. This circularity is mirrored within the play by two key themes: the history of Ned's family relations, discussed in much greater detail in this play than in *The Normal Heart*, and Ned's relationship to various institutional structures, specifically the medical centre where the action takes place and where Ned finds himself the object of a novel treatment. The title of the second play, *The Destiny of Me*, signals the objectification which Ned experiences in the hospital and which is the consequence of Kramer's externalization of self through the production of GMHC and the plays since 'me' as a pronoun can be used both – as it is here – in the possessive case and in the dative or object case.

Brothers and fathers

In both the familial and the institutional context Ned has to fight sameness and difference. Difference is always painful for him. He loves his brother Ben passionately, regarding him as a saviour figure in his fight against their father. But Ben is different from him because he is straight and finds it impossible to regard Ned's homosexuality as anything other than an illness. At one point in *The Normal Heart* Ben and Ned have an argument about this issue[25] culminating in Ned saying: 'I will not speak to you again until you accept me as your equal. Your healthy equal. Your brother' (1987: 1/6, 32) This demand indicates that Ned defines the word 'brother' in terms of equality rather than blood relations. But, as the didascales of *The Normal Heart* have already made clear, 'NED *loves* BEN *more than anyone in the world and his approval is essential to him*' (1987: 1/3, 11) The scene is therefore set for a particular kind of reconciliation, effected, perhaps predictably, through the efforts of another 'brother', Ned's dying lover Felix.

In the re-staging of Ned's relationship with Ben and the brothers' relationship to their father in *The Destiny of Me* it becomes clear that these brothers have an investment – Ned more so than Ben, who says: 'I don't believe anybody makes you do anything you don't really want to' (1993: 47) – in maintaining the paternal corpse, that is the memory of the father, whose presence and absence guarantees their sense of self both in relation to each other and in relation to, and as different from, that figure (see Hope 1997). Both sons felt unsupported by their father, who wanted them to bow to a dominant discourse/authority which victimized them. Ben's experience of anti-semitism at West Point which his father expected him to endure but he refused to put up with, constituted a breaking-point with his father. The father's hatred and violence towards Ned whom he regarded as a sissy and of whose close relationship with the mother he was jealous, created the rift between him and Ned which turned Ned into a fighter. United in their rebellion against the father, the brothers' differences surface when they focus upon each other.

The monolithic authority of the father is then supplanted by the multifarious positions of the various sons; it is the absence of the single deciding figure which creates both a proliferation of alternative discourses such as Ned's and Ben's or Ned's and Bruce's in *The Normal Heart* respectively, or Ned's and Tony the doctor's in *The Destiny of Me*, and a crisis of the relative legitimacy of each of these discourses. In the absence of a clear-cut position, that is a monolithic quasi-paternal one, nostalgia for the father as epitomizing a single viewpoint becomes a way of dealing with the trauma of competing positions, the differences among people one thought of as the same, whether the family or the gay community or 'fellow Americans'. On the familial level this nostalgia manifests itself in the replay of the relationship with the father in *The Destiny of Me* in which the father's inadequacies are explained and also in Kramer's introduction to that play where he states: 'As for my parents' lives, well, there is a difference between tragedy and sadness. I cannot bring myself to see my father as Willy Loman ... I wasn't blaming [my parents]. I was trying to understand what in their own lives made them the way they were and how this affected the lives of their children' (xiii).

Metaphorically the nostalgia for the father, and this is nostalgia for an ideal rather than the actual paternal figure, is constructed both through the desire, present in all of Kramer's writing, that his viewpoint be accepted,[26] and through the need to be integrated into the mainstream.[27] These two are, however, incompatible within a conservative heterosexually invested society. They constitute the enigma of Kramer's desire since he equates sameness (the unachievable) with equality, and difference with inequality. The potential gap between the two positions is bridged in his plays through their dramatic structure and endings. Both *The Normal Heart* and *The Destiny of Me* open in a hospital, in a public space where men are confronted with their

HIV-positive diagnoses. In *The Normal Heart* the public arenas of HIV/AIDS are juxtaposed with the play's epigraph which points to the romantic wish of the normal heart 'to be loved alone', in other words the desire of the individual to be recognized as such. This desire is played out in the central character's relationships specifically with his straight brother and with his lover. However, in *The Normal Heart* all scenes involving Ned's straight brother Ben – with the exception of the final reconciliation scene – take place in Ben's office. As a lawyer Ben is quite literally placed on the side of the law, the 'inheritor' to some extent of the father's position, and the embodiment of the mainstream, whom Ned wishes to persuade of the legitimacy of his own views and self. Ben does not share his father's belligerence towards Ned but rather, in a different version of homophobia, views Ned's homosexuality as an illness. Ironically, or predictably, it is not rational argument or a change of perspective that ultimately prompts Ben's and Ned's reconciliation, and the reconciliation is not staged in Ben's office. It is Ned's lover's emotionally charged appeal to Ben that Ned needs him which initiates their reconciliation.

While the play moves between scenes in public places devoted to the discussions about AIDS and how to organize in relation to it, and private scenes between Ned and his brother Ben and his lover Felix, in which the pervasiveness of AIDS finds expression since no context is AIDS-free, it ultimately moves towards the domestication of AIDS through the use of dramatic conventions which both create closure and recreate a particular form of bourgeois theatre. Significantly, Joseph Papp, who first produced *The Normal Heart* in New York, placed the play in 'the great tradition of Western drama', stating that 'Larry Kramer is the first cousin to nineteenth-century Ibsen' at the heart of whose 'powerful political play' is 'love – love holding firm under fire, put to the ultimate test, facing and overcoming our greatest fear: death'[28]. The love Papp refers to is Ned's love for his lover Felix whom he cares for until Felix dies of AIDS and his love for his brother Ben with whom he is reconciled at Felix's deathbed.[29] The final scene of *The Normal Heart* confirms what is at the heart of the matter, Ned's relationship with his straight blood brother to whom he says, 'you mean more to me than anyone else in the world; you always have' (1987: 1/6, 31). The end of this play then effects a double ending: the 'marriage' between Felix and Ned, and the reconciliation between Ned and Ben. The desire for the 'marriage ceremony', a basically heterosexist convention,[30] signals the desire to belong, to be like, to be the same. This desire for equality, variously reiterated by Ned to Ben within this play, is one which was much debated in another context, that of heterosexual feminism, in the 1970s and 1980s. The main critique of such liberal feminism was that it did not critically interrogate the positions of equality it suggested women should aspire to, in other words it left intact those positions which were constructed as the sources of difference and or as inequality. Additionally, it functioned as a celebration of the achievements of a particular position which in themselves warranted some interrogation. Lastly, it did not question the inherent categorizations into masculine and feminine on which the drive towards equality was based and it took one particular, established position as its point of comparison rather than seeking wholesale change. The same is the case here where Ned and Felix, through their 'marriage ceremony', effectively reproduce the heterosexual marriage ceremony but where, through the death of Felix, this 'marriage' is (a)voided and the heterosexual imperative left intact. What is granted is thus instantly withdrawn and the status quo remains preserved.[31] The play therefore suggests that homosexuals are, after all, not the same as heterosexuals and, importantly, that an embodied position of 'different and equal' is unattainable.

More importantly, in the frame of the play what remains and lasts is not the relationship between Ned and Felix but that between Ned and his brother Ben. The family comes out triumphant – it is what counts. When Felix goes to see Ben to tell him he is ill and that Ned needs him, Ben instantly replies, 'I'm sorry I didn't know you were ill. I'll call him right away' (1987: 69). At the point when Ned is to lose his lover, Ben is ready to contact him again. The death of the lover is in a sense the price for the reconciliation. As Eve Kosofsky Sedgwick (1985) suggested in relation to the nineteenth-century novel, there is a homosocial triangle at work here, but whereas in the nineteenth-century novel the triangle functions as an exchange relationship between men in which the object of exchange is the woman, here the exchange relationship is between a straight and a gay brother and the object of exchange is the gay man's lover and thus, in effect, the embodiment and enactment of homosexuality. For the family relationship to be sustained, the gay relationship has to be transfigured, with the 'outsider', the gay lover, becoming the sacrificial victim necessary for the reconciliation between the blood brothers. Furthermore, the death of the person with AIDS suggests the possibility of the death of AIDS itself, underscored by the notion that abstention from sex – declared by various GMHC members in *The Normal Heart* as impossible since it is what constitutes homosexuality – will aid the process. One might argue that, between the death of the person with AIDS and Ned's imperatives around sexual practice, homosexuality is driven into non-existence.

By the time of *The Destiny of Me* Ned himself is HIV-positive and, in line with the underlying theme of *The Normal Heart*, the family now becomes a much more prominent focus in the narrative of the play. In consequence, the play takes on the traits of conventional bourgeois theatre as opposed to agit-prop in a much more sustained way.[52] The central character still wishes to persuade everybody to be like himself, to become a message queen who may change the world through pointing out its inadequacies. Those inadequacies, however, are not just the inadequacies of 'the system', to use an indeterminate phrase which, through its sheer indeterminacy, becomes depoliticized in the sense of ungraspable and therefore beyond the possibilities of change. 'You do not have to have AIDS to have acquired a system deficient and immune.' (1994: 146). Which system is Kramer talking about here? A personal corporeal system? The state? The state apparatuses? Kramer's plays integrate the personal and the political but they do so in such a way that they become an epiphany of the personal. They seem to suggest, structurally, dramatically and semantically, that the intact (heterosexual) family might be the antidote to AIDS. This is a difficult message to cope with. It is also this position which determines the (in)direction of Kramer's new agit-prop, for in the combat between heterosexuality and homosexuality, homosexuality loses out. Beset by HIV/AIDS, it leads its protagonists (back) to the family[53] which is able to accept them only on pain of death – their, i.e. homosexuals', death. In the final scene between Ned and Ben in *The Destiny of Me*, which is also a reconciliation scene of sorts, Ned celebrates Ben's relationship with his wife by saying, 'you grew to love her. I'm sorry I never really had that. For very long' (1993: 3, 74). This triumph of the heterosexual marital union is then reinforced by the heterosexual brother's survival and by Ned's ultimate affirmation of his dependence on Ben when he says, 'I guess you could have lived without me. I never could have lived without you' (3: 74).

Kramer's plays were written at a time when AIDS seemed to mean death. Their historical context was the sense that governmental indifference promoted genocide amongst those afflicted with AIDS, and that only by refusing silence and by pointing to the rising numbers of people dying from AIDS could the action which might bring about change – properly funded research into a cure – be brought about. In consequence Kramer's plays focus prominently on death, both as a matter of volume and in terms of individuals. Yingling (1991) argues that 'What we encounter in the field of AIDS ... is the political regulation of the body around what is encoded as *the* supremely private site of accommodation to discipline: death' (305). This drive to death as a private and privatizing experience is complemented in Kramer's plays by the overriding focus on the individual and the surviving family. The seemingly redemptive quality of this position obliterates the collective experience of AIDS and the need for that experience to translate itself into action. But, as Yingling maintains apropos the Names Project quilt: 'It allows as well an affirmation of identity not fated to succumb to the traps of affirmative, bourgeois culture in its determination to seal that identity and those meanings in a world of alienation and death. Only in such artifacts may the collective experience of AIDS be encountered, and only in encountering that collective knowledge may the gay and lesbian community continue to become visible to itself as something quite other than the site *par excellence* of social atrophy and alienation' (1991: 307).

Notes

1 The image of the soapbox emphasizes at once the notions of campaigning and of theatricalization or performance.

2 The story of Barbra Streisand's involvement with the play is instructive here (Kramer 1994: 92–3; 396–7).

3 Gilman (1988a) discusses the various ways in which representations of disease facilitate the fear of illness, *inter alia* suggesting: 'in some cases it looms as a threat, controlled only by being made visible' (3).

4 Tax-exemption here figures in the same way as it does for charities in the UK. The resultant issue of having to comply with laws that render tax-exempt organizations toothless through not allowing them to campaign, in consequence of which they increasingly become service rather than lobbying organizations, is one which charities in the UK have had to face as well (see Griffin 1995). Tony Whitehead (1989), founder of the Terrence Higgins Trust in London, discusses the problematic of British AIDS organizations' service role where campaigning might have resulted in more government support. See also Aronowitz (1995: 367–8).

5 An instructive comparison might be made between plays written for theatre and produced in conventional theatre spaces, and 'plays' or performances produced outside such conventional spaces.

6 For an extensive discussion of such effects in other contexts of HIV/AIDS representation, specifically television, see Dubin (1992).

7 Kramer (1994) describes these incidents (339) as part of his point that the large numbers of gay taxpayers in the US should organize collectively to influence public rhetoric which attacks the 'promotion' of homosexuality under the guise of misuse of taxpayers' moneys as if there were no gay taxpayers.

8 Audiences are not, of course, homogeneous and expectations of what one might expect to see on stage will, in consequence, vary. This is evident in different theatre critics' responses to any one performance. When *The Destiny of Me* was performed at the Haymarket Theatre, Leicester, in the autumn of 1993, Robin Thornber stated, 'it's a brave subject for a regional rep to commit to its main stage' while Benedict Nightingale maintained that 'the bite has left [Kramer's] words, and his conflict with the establishment has become a sort of reflexive tic'.

9 At the end of his article about the Springfield affair Bradley (1992) cites a telling

interview with Jean Dixon in which she states that 'her vehement opposition to "The Normal Heart" was motivated in large part because she saw how her older son struggled with his own homosexuality' (370).

10 It is important to make clear that this is *not* an argument against such productions or the production of such visibility but that it is intended, in part, to explain the attacks.

11 In the introduction to *The Destiny of Me* Kramer states: 'I should point out that I have always hated anything that borders on the non-realistic ... Nor have I ever been one to write comfortably in styles not realistic, not filled with facts and figures and *truth*' (1993: xii).

12 This is, in terms of underlying attitude, in complete contrast to Kramer, who writes: 'I consider myself a very opinionated man who uses words as fighting tools' (1994: 145) and who, in his 'message queen' speech, but not only there, repeatedly describes himself as engaged in a war, on the front line, stating: 'If I'm going to go, at least I'm going to go out fighting' (148).

13 All translations by this author.

14 This mirrors Kramer's sense of compulsion, expressed with 'I have no choice' (1994: 146) as he becomes a 'message queen'.

15 The narratives referred to here relate to HIV/AIDS activism and the gay community on the one hand and the personal family relations in the character Ned Weeks's background on the other.

16 The reference to 'individual character' aligns this device with naturalistic theatre where the focus, too, is on the individual.

17 Yingling (1991) maintains that 'postmodern governance is not based in the political representation of subjects under the beneficent gaze of a paternal presence' (295). However, this is in a sense exactly how Kramer constructs the subject's relation to the government and its institutions. Kramer writes for instance: 'The inhuman monster Jesse Helms got an amendment passed that requires all government-funded safe-sex materials to in no way mention, illustrate, or discuss homosexuality or the way gays have sex. Way to stop a plague, America. Thanks, Mom and Dad' (1994: 338).

18 I use the phrase 're-played' here to index the fact that these scenes represent a theatricalized version of Kramer's experiences in GMHC, a revisiting of an *ur*-scene of sorts.

19 For an interesting and pertinent discussion of closetedness and 'outing' see Tyler (1997).

20 In *Reports* Kramer repeatedly points out that the sheer numbers of gay people around – if all were visible and utilized their voting power strategically – mean that if they organized collectively they could achieve change.

21 I take 'clones' here not to be a disrespectful term but to indicate identicalness. It is, perhaps, also worth noting that Bruce in *The Normal Heart* is referred to as a 'gorgeous clone' (1987: 1/1, 3) in appreciation of his good looks.

22 In *The Destiny of Me* Ned, re-telling the story of his attempted suicide while at university, relates his despair: 'Pop's right, of course. I'm a failure. (*Looking at himself in the mirror over the sink.*) You even look like Richard ... I am more my father's child than I ever wanted to be. I've fought so hard not to look like you. I've fought so hard not to inherit your failure. Poor newly-named Ned' (1993: 2, 58).

23 Significantly for Kramer's plays here is another deathbed scene which – if it does not prompt reconciliation – at least promotes a shift in understanding of the characters' histories.

24 'You are forbidden to touch your membrum in self-gratification ... Two bachelors must not sleep together. Two bachelors must not gaze upon each other. Two bachelors who lie together and know each other and touch each other, it is equal to killing

a person and saying blood is all over my hands. It is forbidden ... it is forbidden ... I never stopped hating him' (1993: 3, 66).

25 At one stage Ned demands: 'You've got to say it. I'm the same as you. Just say it. Say it!' to which Ben responds: 'No, you're not. I can't say it' 1987: 1/6, 31).

26 In *The Destiny of Me* Ned says, 'Slowly I became a writer. It suited me. I'd finally found a way *to make myself heard*' (1993, 3, 67; emphasis added).

27 Early on in *The Normal Heart* when Ned and Bruce have an argument about how to campaign around HIV/AIDS and Bruce takes the line that the nature of their sexual practice makes gay men different from other people (one assumes heterosexuals), Ned says, 'I don't want to be considered different' (1987: 1/5, 23).

28 The quotations are taken from prefatory remarks by Joseph Papp in *The Normal Heart*, pages unnumbered.

29 This both follows nineteenth-century literary conventions regarding the power of the presence of death to effect emotional reconciliations and represents a common variation of conflict resolution in contemporary AIDS representation as indicated in the character Tommy's narrative in *The Normal Heart* (1987: 2/9, 43).

30 For a different reading of 'ceremonies of the heart', in this instance of lesbians, see Becky Butler (1990).

31 This is also evident in the conventional representations of masculinity and femininity which are portrayed in the play. Ned asserts for instance that he has his caring side from his mother, 'a dedicated full-time social worker for the Red Cross' (1987: 1/7, 34).

32 Formally *The Destiny of Me* plays with time and space, re-creating the past in the present for example, and simultaneously presenting Ned as an adult and as a child, in ways not particularly associated with naturalist bourgeois theatre, but ideologically it owes much to that theatre form. For a useful recent debate of the meaning of realist conventions in theatre see Diamond (1997).

33 Significantly, when Felix is at one of his lowest points in *The Normal Heart* following his HIV-positive diagnosis, he says, 'I want my mother' (1987: 2/10, 50).

7

Safe and sexy? Lesbian erotica/porn in the age of HIV/AIDS

> there are many who see the body – both as a living cultural form and as a subject of scholarly theorizing – as a significant register of the fact that we are living in fragmented times. (Bordo 1993: 287)

> I must, then, concentrate on lesbian desire and sexual relations between women, the area which still remains the great domain of the untheorized and the inarticulate. (Grosz 1995: 219)

Women in HIV/AIDS discourses

Invisibility has been a major issue for women in general, and lesbians in particular, in the context of HIV/AIDS (Bury, Morrison and McLachlan 1992; Doyal, Naidoo and Wilton 1994; Hogan 1997; Wilton 1997). Writers like Richardson (1987; 1994a; 1994b) and ACT-UP/New York Women and AIDS Book Group (1990) have discussed many of the reasons why this invisibility has persisted, from the alignment of HIV/AIDS with gay men as a 'man's disease', the relatively small numbers of women initially infected, the different rates of HIV infection for women and men, the different types of infection typical for women and men, the issue of transmission routes in women and men, to the underrepresentation of women in HIV/AIDS statistics owing to the diagnostic categories employed, the emphasis on condoms which is not the most immediate concern for lesbians, and the sense, especially in the lesbian community, that lesbian sex is safe sex. Kitzinger (1994) outlined the kinds of women likely to feature in media discourses on HIV/AIDS: 'Woman is white, heterosexual and middle-class. She is everybody's sister, wife, and mother' (95).[1] Servicing sons and husbands with HIV/AIDS as the long-suffering mother and wife, acting as carer,[2] keeping the family together at points of crisis, or, alternatively, functioning as the carrier of the virus as 'innocent victim' or in seductive but debased forms as either the deadly attractive female or the prostitute, women have been the object of very specific iconographies in relation to HIV/AIDS. This iconography has articulated and reproduced cultural constructions of female sexuality as heterosexual and either passive, pleasure-denying, other-centred and 'innocent', or seductive, assertive and dangerous to men. Significantly, the Health Authority safer sex promotion campaigns had no equivalent to the 'Hands campaign for bisexual men' (Field, Wellings and McVey 1997: 62–3) aimed at women. In relation to lesbians in particular Richardson (1994b: 163) has discussed the essentializing definitions underlying their representation in HIV/ AIDS discourses (no drug use; no sex with men; no experience of sexual abuse or rape; actual sexual activity almost unimaginable). These essentializing definitions are also implicit in the ways in which HIV/AIDS health promotion campaigns have projected images of women.

Within lesbian contexts these definitions have been shattered by the emergence of queer and the proliferation of writings on lesbian sex (see Whisman 1993, for example) during the late 1980s and 1990s: 'In urban areas of Britain where the lesbian sub-culture is highly commercialised and club oriented, the 90s decade has heralded the breaking of taboos and the voicing of once-forbidden fantasies. These days words like "dildo", and "fist-fuck" slip easily into casual conversation. Muse on fantasies about domestic bliss, however, and you will be met with discomfort' (Blackman 1995: 189). And Gorna (1996) asserts: 'While the big development for gay men in the 1980s and 1990s is HIV positivity, for lesbians it is sex positivity. The last decade saw the birth of lesbian "porn", of sex clubs, of lesbian sex radicals and overall of a more erotically charged lesbian scene' (352). These changes in lesbian culture have given a new visibility to lesbian sexuality and lesbian sex, and require the interrogation of lesbian sexual practices as they are affected by HIV/AIDS. As Wilton (1997) puts it: 'When AIDS came, it slotted neatly into the pre-existing struggle over sexualized representation' (113). In this chapter I shall analyse how lesbian sex has been represented in lesbian writing in order to tease out some of the problems which arise in that representation in relation to issues of safe(r) sex.[3]

Love and sex

In 1997 Gilman bemoaned the fact that safer sex campaign posters 'refuse to treat sex as sex', sublimating it instead 'into other categories such as "love", because the visual language employed comes from the erotic vocabulary of mass advertising' (112).[4] Wilton (1994; 1997) argued that the eroticization of safer sex campaign material had done little to address women's needs within the HIV/AIDS context for precisely the same reason cited by Gilman: re-circulating erotic mass media images, these campaigns failed to engage with the power structures displayed in the images, and perpetuated stereotypes of hetero-masculine and hetero-feminine sexuality and behaviour which were unlikely to enable women to engage in safer sex. One aspect of this stereotyping was the conflation of sex and love into a scenario of sex as a service by the female to the male, a 'romantic sacrifice of her desires' which is ultimately both dangerous and disempowering to women (see Holland *et al.* 1994a: 67–8).

A similar conflation of the romantic and the sexual is visible in lesbian erotic or pornographic representation.[5] Such representation tends to base the quest for the, or an, object of desire on precisely the combination of emotional attachment and sexual activity famously problematized by Adrienne Rich (1980). Rich discusses the power of convention which informs our choices of love objects. She takes up a point endorsed by psychoanalysis, both classic and feminist, that a woman (the female carer) is women's first love object.[6] For this reason 'heterosexuality is *not* a "preference" for women' because 'it fragments the erotic from the emotional in a way that women find empoverish-ing and painful' (216). The consequence is that patriarchy has to enforce heterosexuality through, among other things, particular forms of heterosex-supportive legislation and 'the ideology of heterosexual romance' (224) which fuses the male demand for satisfaction of his sexual, patrilineal, procreative urge with the promise of emotional as well as sexual fulfilment for the woman.[7] 'Internalizing the values of the colonizer and actively participating in carrying out the coloniza-tion of one's self and one's sex' (225),[8] many women submit to the enforcement of heterosexuality 'in the name of love' and even 'unto death'.[9] They do so because heterosexuality is not presented as a *choice* but as 'compulsory', the 'natural' outcome of a 'normal' woman's psychosexual maturation process. Rich suggests that women are manipulated into heterosexuality through a discourse which exploits and re-directs their emotional needs away from the female to the male. The almost universal representation of women as sexualized bodies available to men in the mass media alone allows little room for querying this discourse.

In parallel with Rich's contentions outlined above I would argue that much lesbian erotica/porn – contrary to the common suggestion (akin to the one made by Rich as regards heterosexuality) that such material, especially anything considered *pornographic*, fragments the erotic and the emotional – utilizes representations of the imbrication of the emotional in the sexual as part of its construction. This serves as a palliative for the more problematic aspects of the material, including obscuring issues around safer sex. Typically, Pat Califia (1988a), an in/famous producer of sado-masochistic material, writes in one of her stories:

> Even when correcting serious misdeeds, Berenice [dominatrix and mother to the primary object of her sexual attention in the story] was not brutal. She loved helplessness, she craved the sight of a female body abandoning all decency and self-control. These things are not granted save in loving trust. Dominance is not created without complicity. A well-trained slave is hopelessly in love with her mistress (67).

Noticeably and predictably, this narrative reproduces the power differences frequently both inherent and enacted in heterosexual relational structures, and central to sado-masochistic scenes. The abandonment of 'all decency and self-control' may be interpreted as a form of sexual liberation but also points to the degrading and exploitative experiences of which characters in these representations frequently are the objects. This particular story, centring on a sado-masochistic mother–daughter relationship, and as such recuperative of the primary love relationship between female carer and dependent infant postulated by psychoanalysis, presents a whole series of incest-taboo-breaking relations in which the emotional ties between blood relations (sisters; mother and daughter; aunt and niece) and the notion that they (therefore?) *care for* and *take care of* each other operate as the legitimating framework for their sado-masochistic activities.[10] Similarly, Califia's (1988b) horrendous story entitled 'The surprise party' legitimates the homophobically framed, sado-masochistic abuse of a lesbian by a group of men, supposedly 'cops', by suggesting not only that she desires violent heterosex but also, by indicating towards the end of the story that these are men who are her friends, giving her a surprise birthday party.[11] These are just two examples of what I perceive to be a common phenomenon in *written*[12] lesbian erotica/porn: the conjunction of the emotional with specific sexual practices. This phenomenon is shared with popular (lesbian) romance, which, according to Janice Radway (1987), in its ideal version presents the heroine as 'emotionally complete and sexually satisfied' (149). The conjunction of the emotional and the sexual raises issues concerning the impact of HIV/AIDS on erotica/porn regarding the articulation of sexuality, the relationship between representation and experience,[13] and the depiction of sexual practices to which I shall now turn.

The silence (?) of lesbian sex

In 'Lesbian sex' Marilyn Frye (1991) writes: 'Lesbian "sex" as I have known it most of the time I have known it is utterly inarticulate. Most of my lifetime, most of my experience in the realms commonly designated as "sexual" has been prelinguistic, noncognitive. I have, in effect, no linguistic community, no language, and therefore in one important sense, no knowledge' (6).[14] The connections Frye makes between inarticulacy, absence of linguistic community, and lack of knowledge[15] are crucial here.[16] They resurface in an interview between Sue O'Sullivan and Cindy Patton (1990) in which Patton links what she calls the 'paucity of sexual imagery for lesbians' (132) with the difficulties of promoting safer sex among lesbians. This constitutes a further invisibility, intra-communal this time, which contributes to the absence of lesbians from representations of HIV/AIDS. I shall return to this point later. For now, I want to ask what Frye means when she talks of lesbian sex as 'utterly inarticulate'. What interests me here is that she made these comments in a context and at a historical moment when there had been a *proliferation* of discourses (see Singer 1993) and texts on lesbian sexuality, many of which – if not most – were written by lesbians. It is thus not exactly the case that lesbian sex is inarticulate. However, as Hogan (1997) points out, 'The new visibility … cannot erase the gendered narratives and assumptions that created women's initial invisibility and stereotypical presentations' (110). The new visibility, in fact, perpetuates those gendered narratives and assumptions.

There are a great many texts depicting lesbian sex. The following two very different examples of such texts serve to make the point. One is a short poem by Suniti Namjoshi, entitled 'I give her the rose':

> I give her the rose with unfurled petals.
> She smiles
> and crosses her legs.
> I give her the shell with the swollen lip.
> She laughs. I bite
> and nuzzle her breasts.
> I tell her, 'Feed me on flowers
> with wide open mouths,'
> and slowly,
> she pulls my head down.

(1991: 25)

The second quotation is from a lesbian pulp fiction novel, first published in the 1950s, Ann Bannon's (1959) *I Am a Woman*: '[Laura] clung wordlessly to Beebo, half tearing her pajamas off her back, groaning wordlessly, almost sobbing. Her hands explored, caressed, felt Beebo all over, while her own body responded with violent spasms – joyous, crazy, deep as her soul. She could no more have prevented her response than she could the tyrannic need that drove her to find it' (93). Both texts depict lesbian sex and they do so in different, yet recognizably conventional ways. Made famous by Gertrude Stein, the rose is a well established euphemism for what Jeanette's mother in Jeanette Winterson's *Oranges Are Not the Only Fruit* (1985) calls 'down *there*'. Such natural imagery is commonly employed in the representation of lesbian sex (Griffin 1993: 135–58). It offers overt resistance to the heterosexist view that lesbian sex might be 'unnatural' while reinforcing the problematic notion that women are somehow closer to nature than men (see McMillan 1982; Haraway 1991). The scene from Bannon's novel presents sexuality as an irrational and irresistible force which, one might argue, in part suggests that the individual woman, so engaged, is incapable of deliberating about her actions, shaping them and taking responsibility, all of which is, of course, crucial for a safer sex context. The scene also renders the protagonist inarticulate: Laura groans 'wordlessly'. Fade-outs, not just, so to speak, of the visual, but also of the verbal, kind are very common in scenes depicting lesbian sex, creating a division between saying and doing, and suggesting that you cannot do it and talk at the same time.[17] It seems not to be the case then, as Frye suggests, that lesbian sex is 'inarticulate'; rather, this articulacy takes particular forms. Frye talks of 'my *experiences* in the realms commonly designated as sexual' (emphasis added); I take this to refer to actual experiences in her personal life. In the face of the proliferation of discourses and texts on lesbian sex, Frye's assertion indicates not only a gap between the private and the public (private inarticulacy *versus* public verbosity) but also a discrepancy between the two: the fact that lesbian sex is visualized and verbalized in cultural production for consumption by a general public does not as a matter of course enhance articulacy in the private sphere. Rather, to judge by the excerpt from *I Am a Woman*, for example, the public description of lesbian sex *reinforces* not only the divide between the public and the private in the realms of sexuality but also the notion of silence during sex in the private context. In her discussion of running safer sex workshops Mary Louise Adams (1988) writes: 'Overcoming squeamishness about dental dams is but the least of our worries' (112). The lack of discussion of sex among lesbians, in private and in public, leads to a situation where 'we live and love in communities that rarely make space for the airing of sexual difficulty or difference' (Adams 1988: 113). In Adams's narrative safer sex becomes the motivation for a 'new terrain for sexual debate … in which we had permission – indeed we were obliged – to talk about sex, graphically, non-judgmentally' (1988: 113). Against the notion that 'lesbian sex "just happens"' (1988: 114), Adams suggests that safer sex requires premeditation and 'implements', a performance diametrically opposed to the images generated in the texts that present lesbian sex which I cited above.

Negotiating safe(r) sex

Namjoshi's poem and Bannon's novel operate within specific cultural and narrative conventions gleaned from romance which include, for instance, natural imagery and the 'speechlessness' of the lesbian protagonists when they engage in sex. The latter convention of constructing action and speech as divorced from each other is particularly important here since that division is one of the concerns in discussions about erotica/porn *per se*, and about erotica and safer sex specifically. The need for safer sex in the age of HIV/AIDS has generated an imperative for a new sociality of sex, for negotiation and communication as the basis of sexual activity. This is evident, for example, in the logocentricity of health promotion campaigns and in slogans these employ such as 'How far will you go before you mention condoms?'[18] The very question points to the need to become articulate in sexual contexts in order to negotiate safer sex but it also points to the problematic of doing so since the sequence of images related to the caption asked repeatedly, 'This far?', 'Or this far?' showing a heterosexual couple going further and further into sexual activity without, implicitly, having got around to discussing the condom issue yet.

The separation of erotic action from protective meta-discourse revealed here resurfaced in lesbian erotica/porn of the late 1980s. This is evident in Sheba Collective's (1989) introduction to *Serious Pleasure* in the assertion of a difference between what is presented as text and what 'real' people do in 'real' life.[19] It also surfaces in the intratextual construction of an articulate, controlling, 'doing' character whose sexual demands are made explicit and the passive, 'done to', silent other who services those sexual demands. The result of this problematic is indicated by Cindy Patton in her interview with Sue O'Sullivan (1990) when she suggests that it is difficult to establish safer sex practices if no discourse about lesbian sex is in circulation in the lesbian community. In discussing the difficulties of trying to create lesbian safe sex discussions, Patton explains: 'What it really felt like was that even lesbians didn't know what it was that lesbians did in sex, so there was no way that we could come up with a formula for figuring out what lesbian safe sex was' (121).

Concerns about the presentation of lesbian sex and its relation to HIV/AIDS have surfaced in the context of lesbian erotica/porn because these depict sexual practices and behaviours which can heighten the risk of HIV infection. That such concerns have surfaced is not to say, however, that lesbians assume a unified position on this matter. In 'Fairy tales, "facts" and gossip: lesbians and AIDS', for example, Tessa Boffin (1990b) cites a variety of lesbians' views on lesbian sex and AIDS, one of which is, 'Lesbians worldwide are not a risk group.[20] Lesbian sex is safe … Only nuns show fewer cases of sexually transmitted diseases than lesbians' (Boffin 1990b: 156). In a parallel essay entitled 'Angelic rebels: lesbians and safer sex' Boffin comments: 'These women [i.e. lesbians who take that stance] also regard us as virgin angels, immune to infection by virtue of the fact that lesbian sex is somehow seen as purer, cleaner and safer than any other form of sexual practice. This view fails to acknowledge that there are certain activities such as rimming, fisting, cunnilingus, and so on, which cut across the fragile boundaries of sexual orientation, and could put anyone, regardless of their sexuality or gender, at risk' (1990a: 57). Boffin's comment points to the arguments among lesbians regarding identity and activity. As Gorna (1996) puts it: 'what is a real lesbian?' (357).

Sexual practices which can heighten the risk of HIV infection and which are associated with sado-masochism, gender bending and queer have generated major divisions among lesbians, partly but not only in generational terms, with the younger generation, to put it crudely, identifying with queer and the older generation viewing themselves as lesbian feminists.[21] All sides tend to avoid engaging with the issue of co-factors (see Vazquez 1998) which are significant in increased risk of HIV infection, seeking instead to focus only on sexual activity. Vazquez (1998) analyses how excluding that position is, often simply reproducing a white, middle-class viewpoint of lesbians and HIV/AIDS. Lesbians, however, do not have one shared identity and set of habits. That is evident even in the range of lesbian erotica/porn available to women. It also remains the case that little women-specific research is done regarding HIV/AIDS (see Hollibaugh 1998).[22] For a variety of reasons lesbians appear to represent a low-risk group in terms of the likelihood of getting infected with the HIV virus (see Leonard 1990; Richardson 1987). However, as Richardson (1994b) makes clear, women are under-represented in HIV/AIDS statistics owing to diagnosis issues, and lesbians are utterly invisible: 'the media coverage has both illustrated and reinforced heterosexist assumptions about women. HIV/AIDS statistics are routinely presented in ways which distinguish between men of different sexual "persuasions" but treat women as an amorphous, single category ... [in which] lesbians are rendered invisible' (Kitzinger 1994: 96).[23] The virus appears to be transmitted through bodily fluids, specifically blood, including menstrual blood and vaginal secretions. Activities that involve such fluids when one partner is infected can put the other person at risk. Being low-risk does not mean that you are immune, and publishers, writers and editors of lesbian erotica/porn have had to, and are having to, respond to the question of how to deal with the issue of HIV/AIDS in the context of the representation of lesbian sex, and whether or not to make the depiction of safer sex practices part of their presentation of lesbian sex.[24] The responses have changed over time, they are revealing, and they indicate why establishing safer sex practices is so problematic.

A question of responsibility?

Alyson Publications, who publish Califia's writings, have, as Califia (1988a) puts it, 'a policy against eroticizing high risk sex' (17), which means that Califia had to re-write any material which included the exchange of bodily fluids. Sheba, who published *Serious Pleasure* (1989), have no such policy. However, in the late 1980s the Sheba Collective who edited *Serious Pleasure* and Califia felt impelled to discuss AIDS and safer sex in the introductions to their respective texts and to include 'Notes on AIDS and safer sex' in the back of their books. Despite Sheba Collective maintaining that 'we do not believe that all fictional writing or visual representation of lesbian sex should immediately incorporate safer sex guide lines' (1989: 12), ignoring HIV/AIDS was clearly not an option.

In their discussions on whether or not to include safer sex practices in representations of lesbian sex, both Califia and Sheba made distinctions between saying and doing, fantasy and reality. Both used this distinction to validate publishing erotica/porn in the same way that feminist critiques of romance have used it to address issues around the 'legitimacy' of popular romance as 'fantasy fodder' for women oppressed within heteropatriarchy.[25] The Sheba Collective wrote:

> *Serious Pleasure* is in no way a lesbian sex manual. In the same way that fantasy is no indication necessarily of what any individual will do in 'real life', neither are the stories in *Serious Pleasure* what either the authors or the readers necessarily 'do'. Safer sex is a case in point. Interestingly none of the stories submitted to us included safer sex as an issue either to be addressed in the context of the story or built into a sexual encounter ... Do lesbians in general still believe that AIDS is not a significant reality for them in terms of sexual transmission? We would guess that this is so and

may be the primary reason for the absence of any mention of safer sex in these stories. (1989: 11–12)

Note Sheba Collective's own conflation of reality and fantasy here: first maintaining that there is no necessary relation between fantasy and reality, they then go on to suggest a direct connection between lesbians' practice outside and in the text. Similarly, and I would suggest without being aware of the ambiguity of her statement, Califia writes: 'Images and descriptions are forever getting confused with live acts' (1988a: 17).[26] Precisely!

This leads me to the issue of the consumer of lesbian erotic/porn and her – and I shall consider only the lesbian consumer here – relation to that material. What does she want from it? Entertainment, escape, education? There does not seem to be a simple answer to this question but it appears to be the case that at least some lesbian readers some of the time go to lesbian erotica/porn for information or education,[27] to gain knowledge about lesbian sex. Jan Brown (1992) illustrates this. If it is the case that lesbian readers read lesbian erotica/porn for information, does this or should this mean that publishers and writers of such material have a responsibility to these members of the lesbian community to provide them with appropriate information concerning safer sex practices?

One could argue about this question in terms of the responsibility a publisher or writer has towards the community whom she serves and lives off. This moves the debate not only into the realm of the economic (to put it cynically and unceremoniously: what profit is there in promoting practices that kill the consumers of your goods?)[28] and, more importantly, into the realm of the ethical. In the late 1980s Sheba Collective and Califia both engaged with the question of the responsibility for providing appropriate information about 'safer sex' and found themselves answering with a qualified 'yes'. As Sheba Collective put it:

We believe that all lesbians should think long and hard about HIV and AIDS and seriously take on the hows and whys of safer sex. For some, erotic stories consciously built around safer sex practices might be helpful. *Serious Pleasure* has not included that possibility in its brief. Even if unprotected lesbian sex was clearly a high risk behaviour we do not believe that all fictional writing or visual representation of lesbian sex should immediately incorporate safer sex guide lines. However, we feel it is important that the issue of safer sex is always acknowledged in some way. We have included some information which you will find at the back of the book. (1989: 12)

What I want to highlight here is not so much the issue of the publisher's/writer's responsibilities as the fact that this issue, it seems to me, can arise only in a context where safer sex and erotica/porn are viewed as two discrete entities, uneasily co-existing as indeed they do in the texts under consideration. The fact that 'Notes on safer sex' are separated out from the erotic/pornographic material which forms the main part of these books suggests a split in cultural consciousness, reiterated in the introductions of *Macho Sluts* and *Serious Pleasure*, between safer sex and sexual practices, which is reinforced by the fact that both are presented as very different forms of discourse, so that the erotic/pornographic texts are encoded in conventional narrative terms whereas the notes on safer sex display the characteristics typical of a discourse one would associate with information or instruction rather than with romance.[29]

The power of convention

I want to consider briefly some explanations for why Califia and Sheba Collective exhibit such reluctance in facing HIV/AIDS and safer sex in their texts. One of these is associated with the earlier distinction between fantasy and reality, and with the fact that depictions of lesbian sex are subject to cultural and narrative conventions. One of the sources of these conventions, romance, demands the construction of an object of love or desire which is perfect in a variety of ways including perfectly healthy – at least initially. To project such an object as – at least potentially – the carriers of STDs (sexually transmitted diseases) raises all sorts of questions about that object's sexual behaviour which would explode the very sexual ideology underlying romance on which the latter is founded.

Additionally, the narrative structure of romance demands a closure which leaves the heroine corporeally and otherwise intact and looking forward to a bright relational future.[30] In terms of specifically literary definitions, romance conforms to the conventions of comedy rather than tragedy – it requires life, not death as its ending (see N. Frye 1973). In western culture, and despite the conventions of Christian mythology which promise a great afterlife (though at the price of a horrible death – witness Jesus on the Cross), death is not something to celebrate. It therefore cannot be a central part of comic or romance conventions. One might argue that the current emphasis on 'living with' rather than 'dying from' AIDS enables the possibility of a re-writing of such texts, a visibilization of HIV/AIDS and safer sex within a context changed by the possibilities of sustained survival. However, not only does romance require life as its ending; it has to be unequivocal. Ambiguity in resolution would be the death of romance; the mere suggestion of safe sex therefore, which of course implies the possibility of death, would raise doubt, uncertainty, concerning the future of the heroine: what would happen if she or her partner was a carrier of HIV? Given the continued uncertainty of its incubation time and of any related diseases,[31] when would we, the readers, be assured that everything was OK? One might thus argue that the inclusion of safer sex practices in lesbian erotica/porn would necessitate a radical revisioning of the construction of such material which could, after all, no longer utilize the formulae of romance as we know them. What is thus interestingly indexed is that on one level at least, lesbian erotica/porn are fantasies, not representations of what lesbians do but presentations of imaginary scenarios in which the reality, namely that even lesbians can get HIV-infected, is displaced in favour of a fantasy that either no matter what we do we cannot catch it, or no matter whether we catch it or not, we do not care.

Safer sex is not 'sexy' in two senses of that phrase: it has not – as yet – been sufficiently conventionalized as part of erotic/pornographic representation, and it is not trendy to think of doing it. The latter may be because, as Gayle Rubin (1988) maintains, 'in times of great social stress ... disputes over sexual behaviour often become the vehicles for displaying social anxieties, and discharging their attendant emotional intensity' (267). In other words, living as we still do in dangerous times, riskier sex, meaning unsafe sex, becomes a way of displacing and discharging those anxieties for which we have no other obvious outlet. It is also the case that we live in a society which displays an overt consciousness of violence, violence that can simultaneously be brought into our homes and is contained – inside the television or video machine. The same is evident in other cultural forms such as the cinema and books. Increasingly, we thus become inured to violence but are also offered the notion that while it occurs, it will not happen to us.[32] A parallel can be drawn to HIV/AIDS. We are thus left with the problematic of how to engage with HIV/AIDS in the context of lesbian erotica/porn. This difficulty clearly surfaces in Califia's writing, which is fraught with contradictions about 'safe' *versus* 'risky' sex. It is also evident in Sheba Collective's stories where 'safe' *versus* 'risky' is frequently negotiated through making explicit that the events depicted are the narrator's fantasies.

Imaging HIV/AIDS

One further element which compounds the difficulties of presentation detailed above is concerned with the imaging of HIV/AIDS. Rejecting 'feminist erotica' Califia writes: 'This stuff reads as if it were written by dutiful daughters who are trying to persuade Mom that lesbian sex isn't dirty, and we really are good girls, after all' (1988a: 13). Sheba in their notes on safer sex maintain: 'Learning about safer sex is a way of collectively talking about what we do sexually. It is also a way of confronting the notion that if you decide to practice safer sex you are "unclean" or suspect your partner of being so' (1989: 200). The words 'dirty' and 'unclean', by association, surface the idea of contamination, illness, and social marginalization.[33] Both Califia and Sheba seem to suggest that if, in doing lesbian sex, we are supposed to be 'dirty' in the eyes of the world or our partner, then at least we want to be able to decide what the nature of the dirt is: Califia seeks to appropriate and re-value the term 'dirt' to index something positive; Sheba are looking to disarm it by questioning its appropriateness. Califia again: 'I don't believe "unsafe" porn causes AIDS ... Nobody ever caught a disease from ... a book' (1988a: 17).

Lesbian erotica/porn, in Califia's book, are sexy (when unsafe) and safe (because only a text). Here we find, inversely expressed, the notion that by not incorporating – and note that word – safer sex practices, by not taking precautions into the body of writing, we might lay ourselves open to disease, that contamination may be the result of unsafe sex. Simultaneously, by taking it in, by incorporating safer sex practices into lesbian erotica/porn, we are taking it, HIV/AIDS, on. Does taking it on mean being contaminated by it? This question, I would suggest, produces another reason why Califia and Sheba Collective are reluctant to include safer sex practices into their erotica/porn, indicating a persistent question and anxiety about how we get it – HIV/AIDS – and what we should do about it.

It might be argued that through the denial of HIV/AIDS, as much as through the incorporation of safer sex practices into lesbian erotica/porn, we are romancing death.[34] A recent example of this occurs in Gayla Mann's (1999) story 'The Scrimshaw butch', which explores s/m relationships. In a scene in which the protagonist's current lover elaborately cuts her with a razor as part of their love-making, the protagonist remembers her former, now dead lover: 'Spread on our four-poster, pelvis up to meet my Danne's fisted thrust, I see the fluid and misty landscape of ecstasy, where the passage of time and death are not real things' (240). As the protagonist engages in what are high-risk activities, she images a state of sexual arousal where 'time' and 'death' are not 'real'. The protagonist is cast as letting go of her former lover through this process, of laying the ghost of that person to rest. But it is also a romancing of death which takes no account of the present and the meaning of those activities as related to time and death. HIV/AIDS does not figure here.

One thing seems clear to me: the emergence of HIV/AIDS has called for a re-visioning of lesbian erotica/porn which is not evaded by avoiding the issue. Lesbian erotica/porn means something different now from what it meant before HIV/AIDS had arrived. One might argue that the proliferation of lesbian erotica/porn since that period (witness the revival of *on our backs*, a queer pornographic magazine) has made a re-visioning all the more necessary. It is possible that the proliferation of this material constitutes an act of defiance, a refusal to be beaten by the public discourses around the disease, not all of which are terribly accurate and many of which are homophobic. It could also be a romancing of death which resembles that associated with the decadence of the 1890s when 'living for the moment' supplanted the orientation towards a future many no longer believed in (see, for example, Showalter 1991, especially chapters nine and ten). Sarah Lucia Hoagland (1988) has called for a revaluing of lesbian desire which states that such desire need not be 'a matter of being "safe" or "in danger"', but is 'a matter of connection' (169). She asserts: 'Thus we can come to embrace more fully both desire and difference as biophilic, not necrophilic' (169–70). The question of course is: who or what do we connect with? And how?

Since uncertainty prevails, the visibility of HIV/AIDS in lesbian erotica/porn has changed during the 1990s. I would suggest that concerns with HIV/AIDS have, in fact, become less visible. They are invisible in *Best Lesbian Erotica 1999* (Taormino 1999), for instance. As detailed above, in 1988 Califia felt compelled to produce two parallel discourses – the one pornographic, the other informational, to give safer sex practices a place in her text. But by 1993 the nature of the second discourse had begun to change.[35] In *Melting Pot* Califia (1993) includes a final section, 'Slipping', consisting of a series of anecdotes which portray lesbian and gay life and sex in the age of AIDS. Intended not as fiction but as a presentation of 'reality' as we live it now, it reveals the ambivalences and contradictions which lesbians and gay men face in this age. A number of key points emerge. They include:

- the notion that 'lesbians have AIDS envy' (207) since they talk about safer sex when HIV/AIDS isn't really a problem for them
- the difficulty of using dental dams effectively, the absence of research on their effectiveness, and the consequent non-use of such dams, even at safe sex parties for leatherwomen
- the relative lack of information about lesbians' risk of HIV infection

- the continuing debate about what is a 'real' lesbian and the notion that 'if a woman has AIDS, she must not be a real lesbian' (210)
- the differential ways in which safe sex information for lesbians and straight men is constructed though both have sex with women (e.g. straight men are not advised to use dental dams when going down on a woman)
- lesbians engaging in s/m are more likely to articulate and negotiate sexual practices than 'vanilla' lesbians and therefore possibly less at risk from HIV infection ('Women who refuse to talk to S/M dykes don't seem to want to talk to each other about AIDS' (213)).

Califia states that 'my track record with safer sex is less than perfect' (222)[36] and reiterates the notion that sex is a force which voids those in its grip of the ability to deliberate: 'We slip because the condition of being aroused creates moisture. Hazardous footing. Melts boundaries. Makes the edges fuzzy. Creates immediate needs that overwhelm our ability to plan for the future' (1993: 223). Caught between the continuing lack of knowledge about lesbians and HIV/AIDS and the conventions governing representations of sex and romance, Califia in 'Slipping' charts a map of the ambiguities which inform the presentation of contemporary lesbian and gay sex lives. Disturbing and seemingly honest at the same time, her text indicates that visibility does not in and of itself offer solutions to the problems of how to be a sexually active lesbian in the 1990s.

Whilst Califia writes about the ambivalences that HIV/AIDS has created in lesbian and gay life, Gorna (1996) takes a line which is in part condemnatory of lesbians as attempting to 'get in on the act' of HIV/AIDS. Her critique of lesbian involvement in safe/r sex issues focuses on 'latex lesbianism', 'an approach which advocates a range of latex barriers to prevent HIV' (338) which she regards as promoted in particular by 'the producers of lesbian porn' (353). She both tells the reader that there is a hypothesis that 'the lesbians who overemphasize the possibilities of "woman-to-woman transmission" are suffering from "AIDS envy"' (350) and states that those promoting latex 'do not have "AIDS envy"' (374). However, she offers three basic reasons (357) why latex lesbianism has come into being:

1 It is a way of (re)claiming lesbian sexual visibility and sex positivity, derived from the notion that '[Lesbian] sex is so real it can even be life-threatening' (357).
2 It is a way of avoiding bodily fluids, described by Gorna as 'the "yuck!" factor' (355).

3 'It can even become an excuse for being upfront' (357), for talking about sex.

Gorna makes many important points in her text but these three reasons offered for the (in her view in the main wrong-headed) promotion of safe/r sex among lesbians strike me as silly. Lesbian sexual visibility has relied on many encodings over the last ten years, of which latex may well be the least important. Indeed, as Califia's 'Slipping' makes clear, latex in the narrow sense of dental dams is slipping out of view. To suggest that the idea of latex lesbianism becomes a way of making sex more 'real' because life-threatening assumes that sex is significant or exciting only if life-threatening, a position which may hold attractions for some – but, I would suggest, a relatively small number of lesbians. This point is reminiscent of the AIDS envy view referred to by both Califia (1993) and Gorna of which I am not convinced, despite Gorna's presentation of 'Munchausen AIDS' among lesbians (369–71). Finally, the notion that HIV/AIDS somehow legitimates talking about sex is contradicted by the fact that as regards lesbian erotica/porn there is plenty of talk about lesbian sex and not much, if any, about safe/r sex.

One of Gorna's key points is that assessing the relativity of risk is important for getting to grips with the safe/r sex needs of given individuals. This is undoubtedly the case. But the history of lesbian erotica/porn of the last ten years as indexed in the sample discussed in this chapter suggests that the continuing lack of information about the impact of HIV/AIDS on lesbians has (re-)invisibilized safe/r sex and HIV/AIDS among lesbians rather than promoting more informed writing within the erotica/porn context, for example. HIV/AIDS seems to have gone back into a closet shared only by those lesbians directly involved with HIV/AIDS activism, or those who know people suffering from HIV/AIDS.

Notes

1 This is evident, too, in the portrayal of women in Kramer's theatre and in Kay's poetry related to HIV/AIDS, especially in *The Adoption Papers*.

2 See Bury *et al.* (1992); Dorn *et al.* (1992); Schwartz (1993); Roth and Fuller (1998), esp. chapters 7 and 8.

3 I use 'safe(r) sex' here to indicate the issue of risk elimination (= safe sex) versus risk reduction (= safer sex) which has informed debates about HIV/AIDS. Gorna (1996: 344) discusses this issue in relation to lesbian communities, and what she constructs as a kind of hysteria among certain lesbians regarding safe(r) sex.

4 Holland *et al.* (1994b) discuss the ways in which masculine sexuality in a heterosexual context is achieved through the separation of sex and love, activity and emotion.

5 I shall not rehearse arguments about what constitutes the erotic or the pornographic

here. I find unsatisfactory the subtleties around mutuality versus one-way interactions, whole-body versus bit-part presentations etc. as argued over in essays such as Gloria Steinem (1980) or Audre Lorde (1980). I agree with Gayle Rubin's (1988) assertion that 'Most people find it difficult to grasp that whatever they like to do sexually will be thoroughly repulsive to someone else, and that whatever repels them sexually will be the most treasured delight to someone, somewhere ... Most people mistake their sexual preferences for a universal system that will or should work for everyone' (283). In line with Rubin's position, I would also argue that those who distinguish between erotica and porn frequently do so on the basis of what they find un/acceptable: the acceptable is erotic, the unacceptable is pornographic. I shall therefore use 'erotic/pornographic' throughout the chapter.

6 In a pertinent discussion, towards the end of *Bodies that Matter* (1993: 230–42) and subsequently in *The Psychic Life of Power* (1997), Judith Butler develops an argument according to which the disavowal of that first love object generates gender performance and 'allegorizes a loss it cannot grieve [the loss of the first love object]' (1993: 235).

7 In her elaboration of the argument that the loss of the primary love object generates gender melancholia Butler (1997: 132-59) discusses not only heterosexual femininity but also heterosexual masculinity as a performance consequent upon the foreclosure of certain kinds of attachment, specifically homoerotic ones.

8 Holland *et al.* (1994a: 65–8) produce a striking example of this in their research on young women's understanding of sexual intercourse as being penile penetration of the vagina, with the primary object of enabling the male to have an orgasm.

9 Extensive research on domestic violence has demonstrated, *inter alia*, that women 'read' men's violence towards them as an expression of their emotional commitment and find it difficult to leave men who are violent, even if their life is in danger. This problematic is exacerbated by the fact that leaving a violent man does not necessarily end the violence or the persecution (Radford and Russell 1992).

10 The same legitimating framework is frequently used in cases of child sexual abuse and other forms of domestic and institutional sexual abuse.

11 The conventionality of this type of narrative closure in erotica/porn for women is demonstrated in the introduction to *Herotica 6* (see Sheiner 1999: viii) where Shreiner states, 'Admittedly, some of these stories employ the old "Surprise, I knew him all along!" ending, but that was inevitable' (x). Importantly, it foregrounds the role of those close to the object of the s/m scene as the 'perpetrators'. This replicates the fact that sexual and other abuse is frequently committed by those close to the victim.

12 Written and visual material needs to be distinguished here, not least because visual material that presents more than one person does not as a matter of course make explicit the relational connections between the people it depicts though it is often very explicit in its presentaton of a particular and unequal power dynamic.

13 This is not to suggest that experience is unmediated but, rather, that the relationship between representation and experience constitutes a contested terrain.

14 M. Frye is not alone in this assertion. Richardson (1994b: 160) points to taboo issues in lesbian communities which include 'talking about the kinds of sex women have together'. See also Roth and Hogan (1998).

15 Valverde (1985) includes a pertinent chapter tellingly entitled 'Lesbianism: a country that has no language'.

16 For another version of this problematic see Kitty Tsui's (1992) 'Who says we don't talk about sex?' in which she considers the impact of her Chinese upbringing on her initial inarticulacy about sex, commenting, for instance: 'Chinese is my first language. But I was fluent only in the words deemed necessary for me to know. I was certainly

not taught the words for breast, cunt, ass, or orgasm. There were no words for sex; therefore sex did not exist' (385).

17 This is a convention much exploited in hetero pulp romances aimed at a female audience such as those published by Harlequin or Mills and Boon, or Barbara Cartland's which typically move from dialogue to euphemistic description at the point of the depiction of actual sexual intercourse as in: '"I love ... you! I love ... you!" she wanted to say, but the Earl was carrying her up on a shaft of moonlight into the sky' (Cartland 1987: 140). The idea seems to be to establish sex as belonging to the realm of the pre-linguistic, a 'pre-social', instinctual phenomenon enacting an inherited 'natural' behaviour. It also suggests automatic sexual response and success, the partner always knowing what you want and fulfilling that desire. All of this is of course consummately contradicted by the reports on sexuality which became in/famous from the late 1940s onwards and which chart, *inter alia*, women's frustration in heterosex (see Jeffreys 1990, esp. chapters two and three).

18 Sadly, the HEA never saw fit to issue an ad with the caption, 'How far will you go before you mention dental dams?'

19 Such splitting between textuality and actuality is frequently used to produce cultural material which exceeds what is perceived to occur 'actually', and to legitimate that excess.

20 Clearly, this depends on how you define 'risk group'. A lesbian may be and do many things beside identifying herself as lesbian. Part of her lesbian identity may involve sexual practices that carry a risk of infection. But she may also engage in other practices such as needle sharing, or she may be the recipient of infected blood products, or she may have paid sex with men, all of which can place her at risk (see Richardson 1994b).

21 A somewhat different perspective emerges in an article in *Diva* (Kemp 1999) in which – carefully chosen – lesbians from different generations have their say. They debunk the cliché of the younger, queer and the older, lesbian feminist lesbian alluded to in my text.

22 The overwhelming focus in HIV/AIDS research regarding women – as any cursory perusal of *The Lancet*, for example, will show – is on mother-to-child transmission and on prostitutes.

23 This pattern is repeated in many HIV/AIDS information contexts. The Australian group Positive Women Victoria Inc. run a website entitled 'Women like us' about women infected with the HIV virus. Their images and texts do not refer to lesbians. They state, quite rightly, 'Any woman can get infected with HIV and develop AIDS'. But they then go on to talk about issues around reproduction ('Can you still have a baby?'), and ask, 'Does your partner/husband have AIDS?', followed by, 'Some of us are married or have boyfriends or girlfriends who also have HIV ...'. The intention is, presumably, to treat every woman in an equal way but the effect is to make lesbians at best marginal, at worst invisible.

24 The same is, of course, true for any other representation of sex and, as a quick review of depictions of sex across a whole range of mass media will make clear, at the representational level safer sex issues have simply not been taken on board. To give just one example: gay writer Alan Hollinghurst's latest offering, *The Spell* (1999), features plenty of sex and recreational drug use but not safe sex. HIV/AIDS seems to have gone underground here except as a reference to people who have died.

25 See, for instance, Fowler (1991); Taylor (1989); Radford (1986); Sarsby (1983).

26 That confusion also manifests itself in the introduction to *Herotica 6* (Shreiner 1999) in which the editor simultaneously maintains that 'this is fiction, and we don't know what, if anything, is based on real experience' (ix) and that the stories 'delve into real life experiences' (xi).

27 In the introduction to *Herotica 6* Shreiner (1999), for instance, writes that 'women were looking for stories that would serve to enhance their sexual relationships with long-term partners – stories that might give hints on how to keep the home fires burning beyond The Seven Year Itch, Lesbian Bed Death, kids, careers and hectic schedules' (vii).

28 Some would, of course, argue that women in general and lesbians in particular appear to die only in small numbers from AIDS.

29 This is reminiscent of the split between the sex education girls tend to receive (all biology, penetration and pregnancy) and their experience of the reality of sexual activity. As Holland *et al.* (1994a) describe it, there is 'a particular slant to sex education: too little, too late, too mechanical' (65). Sex education, according to them, 'lacks almost any content on emotions, sexual relationships or female desire' (1994b: 65).

30 Mandy Merck (1993) offers an account of the way in which AIDS and the person who has it can be assimilated and subjected to the conventions of hetero romance in order to affirm the latter.

31 The convention has become to say that the incubation period is approximately ten years (Bury *et al.* 1992: 17).

32 Paradoxically, it is of course women in the home who tend to suffer violence from those at home with them (Radford and Russell 1992).

33 Based on Kristeva (1982), Zivi (1998) offers a sustained analysis of the treatment of people with HIV/AIDS and the construction of subjectivity within a framework of abjection. See also Stacey (1997: 65–96).

34 Judith Butler (1992) discusses the function of 'death' in current debates on the relationship of the politics of 'life and death' in the context of homosexuality and AIDS.

35 I shall not discuss the pornographic texts in this collection in any detail. But I want to mention one story entitled 'Unsafe sex' as it constructs a gay man in a long-term relationship seeking out unsafe sex as an antidote to the stability and safety of his home situation. He, rather than the man engaging in casual sex whom he seeks out, is presented as the threat to the gay community. This constitutes, of course, the opposite scenario to the one Kramer envisages in his pleas for committed relationships (see Chapter 6).

36 This reflects Gorna's (1996) point that 'it is not clear whether many lesbians actually put these ideas into practice' (354). However, it should be seen in a context where extensive exhortation to use condoms has not resulted in significant increases in condom use among heterosexuals (see Chapter 3). It would appear that there continues to exist a major discrepancy between what is preached and what is practised, and not just amongst lesbians or s/m dykes.

Conclusion: what matter bodies?
Philadelphia and beyond

Whatever happened to the plague? (Channel 4 documentary 1999)

Like the fantasy of erotic desire which frames love, the distortions of forgetting which infect memories, and the blind spots laced through the visual field, a believable image is the product of a negotiation with an unverifiable real. (Phelan 1993: 1)

The uncertainties of HIV/AIDS

If 'a believable image' is 'the product of a negotiation with an unverifiable real' as Phelan suggests, then the question of belief, and what one wishes to believe in becomes all the more important, for believability is a function not just of the 'truth' of an image *per se* but of someone's desire to believe that particular image. Images, as indicated in the previous chapters, are subject to conventions, conventions of what a society encourages to be seen and what it suppresses from sight on the one hand, and conventions governing different kinds of representation on the other. These are the 'distortions' of cultural shaping which 'infect' and inform sites of knowledge, collaborating with and encouraging the beliefs that we invest in. As Phelan (1993) so aptly puts it: 'learning to see is training careful blindness' (13). That blindness may be involuntary, that is arise from a lack of knowledge for example, or it may be a studied indifference, the denial of something which is disavowed.

I raise this because it seems to me that the gap, between those directly affected by and fighting with HIV/AIDS and those whose information about HIV/AIDS is derived solely from the mass media, has grown immeasurably since the early 1990s. HIV/AIDS remains a major catastrophe for millions of people but the 'general public' in the UK today is, I think, largely unaware of this. By that I mean that the range of images of HIV/AIDS across diverse visual cultural sites which we were offered in the late 1980s and early 1990s, and which demanded engagement with HIV/AIDS, has receded into fringe theatres, sexual health centres, voluntary and statutory sector organizations dealing with HIV/AIDS, the inside and back pages of newspapers and away from mainstream television and cinema so that one might well ask, lack of knowledge or studied indifference? And: what matter bodies? For the numbers of those with HIV and dying from AIDS-related diseases are truly frightening (Table 1).

Table 1: Global summary of HIV/AIDS epidemic, December 1998

Total no. of people newly infected with HIV in 1998	5.8 million
Total no. of people living with HIV/AIDS	33.4 million
Total no. of people who died from AIDS in 1998	2.5 million
Total no. of AIDS deaths since the beginning of the epidemic	13.9 million

Adapted from UNAIDS/WHO (1998). It is unclear how 'beginning' is used here since HIV/AIDS is difficult to date (see Chapter 4).

In this conclusion I want to explore some of the reasons why HIV/AIDS seems to have receded from public consciousness in this western country, the UK, from the late 1990s, and I shall use the mainstream film *Philadelphia* which came out in 1993 as a liminal text, pointing both to the history of how HIV/AIDS has been treated and to its future as one of continued marginalization and othering. I shall suggest that among the many reasons why HIV/AIDS has vanished from sight, as far as the 'general public' is concerned, are:

● the continuing uncertainties and lack of knowledge around HIV/AIDS
● the initial locating of HIV/AIDS in the gay community and so-called Third World or developing countries which led to an 'othering' of HIV/AIDS among those unaffected that has never been superseded
● the establishment of voluntary and statutory organizations dealing with HIV/AIDS which generate a sense that HIV/AIDS is 'taken care of'
● the 'failure' of HIV/AIDS to take hold in mainstream western communities as initially predicted
● the shift of 'dying from' to 'living with' HIV/AIDS through changes in treatment regimes, and the 'discovery' of people immune to HIV/AIDS despite repeated exposure

- the 'normalization', indeed domestication, of loss and mourning through their repeated enactment in public and private
- 'competing' narratives of ravishment and catastrophe which are given more media space than HIV/AIDS
- the shift from the notion of a single global epidemic to one of multiplicity with its consequent result of fragmentation of effort and political will to effect change.

As Oppenheimer and Reckitt (1997), reporting on the Acting on AIDS conference held in London in 1996 and organized by the Institute of Contemporary Arts and the Terrence Higgins Trust, point out: 'The Acting on AIDS conference made one thing more clear now than ever: fifteen years into the epidemic, there is no progressive consensus about which issues are most urgent, or on how best to strategize HIV prevention and treatment' (3).

Attempting to describe 'The Physical Effects of HIV Disease on Women' Bury (1994) created a text symptomatic of the experience of HIV/AIDS over the last fifteen years or so. She states:

> HIV infection *mostly* follows the same pattern in men and women. *Between a few days and a few months* after infection, *around* the time that the HIV antibody test becomes positive, there *may* be a short illness like flu or glandular fever … This 'seroconversion illness' is *only* experienced by a *minority* of those who become infected. People with HIV infection then remain well for *some* years before developing symptoms of HIV disease. Early symptoms *include* … AIDS … is diagnosed once one of *a number of* conditions has developed, such as … Studies on gay men *suggest* that *on average* it takes ten years for someone with HIV infection to develop AIDS …; that is, 50 per cent of men will develop AIDS within ten years of infection with HIV while 50 per cent of men with HIV infection will take *longer than ten* years to develop AIDS. Similar research *has not been done* on drug users or on women with HIV infection so at the present time it is *not possible* to say how long it takes for a woman with HIV infection to develop AIDS. (35–6; emphasis added)

This text may date from 1994 but its content remains valid. I quote it at length to reveal some of the difficulties writers on HIV/AIDS encounter as they attempt to be precise about the knowledge bases we have for HIV/AIDS. Bury is trying to be accurate in this account, and to give the best information she can, but, as the italicized sections of the text indicate, much of what she writes about is fraught with uncertainties, incomplete or non-existent information, and redolent with qualifications which relativize the specificity of the knowledge provided. The lack of knowledge visibilized here reflects a wider, continued ambiguity about HIV/AIDS. Writing about the same issue, HIV infection in women, some years later, Gorna (1996) states: 'It is not at all clear who these women are, and in terms of their sexual orientations or identities no one even hazards a guess' (96). Such lack of knowledge has promoted the proliferation of discourses around HIV/AIDS since, in the absence of certainty, the discursive field is (virtually) anybody's to inhabit. And, as indicated in my discussion of some of the controversies around HIV/AIDS which have arisen (see in particular Chapter 4),[1] the proliferation continues. Over the years it has become increasingly clear that HIV/AIDS refuses to be identified with particular groups of people, and that the behaviours associated with 'high risk activities' are not specific to any one group of people, stereotypes notwithstanding. Attempts to map HIV/AIDS have proved problematic and so have predictions of epidemiological developments. Few will now even remember that in 1983 the World Health Organization asserted that AIDS posed 'no risk to the public at large' (McGregor 1983)[2] but it forms an interesting contrast with an article which appeared in *The Observer* only one year later, in 1984, stating that the 'AIDS battle is being lost' (McKie and Timbs 1984). Such veering between denial and assertion has remained a constant aspect of HIV/AIDS debates.[3] Indeed, from a situation where – in the UK – rapid rises in figures of those with AIDS were predicted in the 1980s we are now in a situation where, in January 1999, Channel 4 ran a television documentary entitled 'Whatever happened to the plague?', the title clearly serving as an index of the idea that the panic about the AIDS epidemic which was much heralded in the press in the mid-1980s, around the time of the death of Rock Hudson,[4] has abated to the point of HIV/AIDS becoming invisible (again). AIDS may still be the 'world's number one killer infection' (Lean 1999) but in Britain today we hardly notice it any more.[5] If we have not seen it for a while ('whatever happened to ...?'), maybe it has not been around.[6] Those unaffected by HIV/AIDS seem to have developed the 'careful blindness' Phelan refers to (1993: 13). For them HIV/AIDS appears to be a thing of the past – almost; it does not seem present, and its place in our future, if it has one, is uncertain, to say the least. Historically, what appears to have happened is that we have moved from 'dying from AIDS' to 'living with AIDS', with all the concomitant effects this has produced in cultural representation.

Performance and/as disguise in *Philadelphia*

One visual text which is poised between the notions of dying from and living with HIV/AIDS is the US film *Philadelphia* (1993). It forms part of what Butler (1993) in *Bodies that Matter* refers to as 'the increasing theatricalization of political rage in response to the killing inattention of public policy-makers on the issue of AIDS' (233). This theatricalization, a process of making visible through performance, manifested itself in a whole range of cultural productions around HIV/AIDS, some of which I have already discussed in this volume. Jonathan Demme's *Philadelphia* is one of the productions which achieved mainstream status, evidenced, for instance, in the fact that the film gained its lead actor Tom Hanks an Academy Award as Best Actor. But, as I shall indicate, it did so in part by articulating a moral economy which is fundamentally conservative and, indeed, homophobic, ultimately relegating HIV/AIDS to a secondary position relative to homosexuality, which is the key concern of this film.

At issue in *Philadelphia* are a variety of performances which test the uncertain borders of identity and the grounds on which inclusion and exclusion within specific hegemonic orders are produced. The film's narrative centres on the character of Andrew Beckett, a young gay lawyer suffering from AIDS-related illnesses who is made senior associate in a prestigious firm of lawyers only to be fired when the senior partners, whilst alleging poor professional performance as the motive for sacking him, discover that he has AIDS. Beckett has kept quiet, that is performed heteronormativity and health, at work regarding both his homosexuality and his HIV-positivity because of the homophobia of the senior partners. The film vindicates his choice to remain silent by revealing their prejudices as the motivating force behind Beckett's dismissal. It makes clear that at stake in the senior partners' behaviour is not Beckett's illness but his homosexuality, of which the marks of AIDS, the lesions on Beckett's face, 'simply' become the outward sign.

Beckett is presented as a star performer in terms of his professional and his personal identity. He is a successful lawyer and he passes successfully in the homophobic environment of his professional life. But the provisionality of these identities is exposed when his work is sabotaged by the deliberate misplacement of an important file (thus undermining his professional performance) which becomes the immediate ground for his dismissal, and his ability to pass is threatened when he develops KS (Kaposi's sarcoma) lesions on his face which he is unable to hide despite attempts to do so through using make-up. It is thus his body which 'betrays' Beckett to the senior partners and which leads to his being fired. The illusion of a unitary identity integrating professional competence and assumed heterosexuality,[7] on the basis of which the senior partners promoted him, is shattered by the marks on Beckett's body which exceed their meaning as a kind of cancer to point to his homosexuality.

Butler (1997) describes gender as an effect of melancholia in which 'the accomplishment of an always tenuous heterosexuality' manadates 'the abandonment or, perhaps more trenchantly, *preempting* the possibility of homosexual attachment, a foreclosure of possibility which produces a domain of homosexuality understood as unlivable passion and ungrievable loss' (135) for heterosexuals. Butler suggests that 'this heterosexuality is produced ... by enforcing the prohibition on homosexuality' (135). Out of this, masculinity (and femininity) emerges as an accomplishment rather than a disposition, something that is arrived at through an active process rather than being innately or latently present. It leads to 'a cultural logic whereby gender is achieved and stabilized through heterosexual positioning, and where threats to heterosexuality thus become threats to gender itself' (135). Beckett posits such a threat to the senior partners in his law firm. Since 'in a man, the terror of homosexual desire may lead to a terror of being construed as feminine, feminized, of no longer being properly a man, of being a "failed" man, or being in some sense a figure of monstrosity or abjection' (Butler 1997: 136), masculinity is strengthened through the repudiations of homosexuality it performs (140). As Butler puts it: 'What cannot be avowed as a constitutive identification for any given subject position runs the risk not only of becoming externalized in a degraded form, but repeatedly repudiated and subject to a policy of disavowal' (1997: 149). This is, effectively, how homosexuality and Beckett are treated in *Philadelphia*.

Beckett attempts to continue his performance as not gay by attempting to conceal the lesions on his face through the use of make-up. As Phelan, writing about performance, suggests: 'performance keeps one anchor on the side of the corporeal (the body Real) and one on the side of the psychic Real' (1993: 167). He utilizes his body to enact an identity he does not, in fact, identify with. This in itself indicates the provisionality of his performance or, more accurately, of *this* performance. The senior partners regarded Beckett as one of their own but the inadvertent discovery of his homosexuality through the visibility of the lesions indicates the return of the repressed or disavowed into their midst, the destabilization of their identities and norms through the hitherto successful passing of Beckett. If he is gay what does that say about them? Homosexuality thus becomes the focus of the film as its denial or assertion demands of those who regard heterosexuality as the norm that they consider their own positions. To adapt a phrase from Butler (1993): 'This is a performative enactment of "[sexuality]" that mobilizes every character in its sweep' (185). This is made clear by Beckett's lawyer in the courtroom not only by pointing it out directly but also, and in consequence, by repeatedly asking various characters if they are gay or homosexual. Their negative responses and blustering repudiations signal the production of homosexuality as the socially abject. Simultaneously, these responses point to the provisionality of the various characters' identities which need to be reinforced through disavowal and abjection. Within this economy, jokes and jibes, such as those articulated by the senior partners at various points in the film, function as the discursive testing ground of their heterosexual identity, (re)asserted through the laugh that abjects that which is joked about.

The senior partners' intolerance of otherness is made manifest in the courtroom scenes through the reports of their treatment of women and of people from diverse ethnic groups. It encourages Beckett to dissociate himself from his homosexuality through the performance of silence. Beckett neither lies nor protests – he lets matters pass. This performance guarantees his inclusion in the inner circle as it affirms by omission the heteronormativity which governs the partners' behaviour and discursive interactions. Once his homosexuality is discovered, the senior partners' perception is that their heteronormativity can be (re)asserted only through abjecting Beckett, thus getting rid of what he stands for. His dismissal is intended to maintain their illusion of heteronormativity by clearly delineating a border between them and him. He is no longer on the inside, that is in their assorted inner sanctums such as their clubs, suites, locker rooms but now exists on the outside, physically separated from them through expulsion from his office. Beckett's dismissal is intended to act as the guarantor of the senior partners' heteronormativity. And, as was the case with Kramer's theatre and with Kay's poems in *The Adoption Papers*, this heteronormativity – which itself becomes the guarantor of mainstream cultural production – is filmicly sustained and affirmed through Beckett's death, the final abjection of the unwanted body which as a particular form of closure promotes the mainstreaming of the film.

'Dying from' versus 'living with' AIDS: unmasking heteronormativity

The film makes this position quite clear through the juxtaposition of Beckett as an AIDS sufferer with Mrs Benedict, a married woman and mother of two who contracted AIDS through a blood transfusion when she lost a lot of blood while giving birth to her second child. Mrs Benedict is constructed as an innocent victim whose illness is not, as articulated in the film, the result of 'reckless behaviour' on her part.[8] She becomes the key witness in asserting that at least one of the senior partners, with whom she worked, knew that KS lesions signify AIDS[9] since she had such lesions as a consequence of her own HIV infection. Mrs Benedict has had lesions on and off for several years and at the point of the trial it is some years since she worked with the partner in question but she is obviously not close to death. In court she is presented as a healthy-looking and compassionate figure who is clearly surviving and does not seem much impaired by her illness. Unlike Beckett, Mrs Benedict has not been dismissed from her job and, more significantly in terms of the heteronormative economy of this film, she is not dying from AIDS but living with it. However, if Beckett is dying why isn't she? Since she is presented as part of the heteronormative world which the senior partners, and I would argue the film, seek to maintain, over-invested in that scenario as 'wife-and-mother', she poses no threat to that world and does not disturb the boundaries of sexual difference it constructs in the way that Beckett is perceived to do. The film's manipulation of this figure to maintain heteronormative boundaries becomes evident when one considers that, whilst it is presented in a realist mode which suggests verisimilitude, the progress of Mrs Benedict's HIV infection is in question through her continued good health *despite* having suffered from KS.[10] To look at Mrs Benedict you would not think she has AIDS. But research on western white women with HIV/AIDS indicates that women are diagnosed later as being HIV-positive and (possibly therefore) die sooner from AIDS-related conditions (Bury 1994; Richardson 1994a). Mrs Benedict's seemingly continued good health and 'failure' to die is thus strikingly at odds with what research on women with HIV would suggest. Where in Beckett's case the KS lesions are made to signal the beginning of his physical decline and death, in Mrs Benedict's case the KS lesions seem to constitute merely an interlude in her general state of well-being with no visible long-term consequences for her health. One might argue that this simply testifies to the diversity of experience of HIV/AIDS which has been asserted throughout this book but one might also ask why Beckett is not juxtaposed with another gay character working in a law firm, for example. Within the world constructed by the film homosexuality is in fact firmly contained both in individual characters (as opposed to proliferating revelations of gay presences across a range of law firms, for instance) and gay-specific sites (Beckett's fancy dress party; the gay porn club referred to in the trial). Indeed, the issue of homosexuality is uncovered only to be masked again through the discourses around HIV/AIDS on which the trial is based, and by keeping homosexuality firmly in its place – on the outside. Through the choice of Mrs Benedict as Beckett's AIDS foil the film affirms both that HIV/AIDS does not discriminate among bodies *and* that it is still possible to differentiate between them since bodies signal more than their physical materiality (Grosz 1994: xi), and it is that *more* which is at stake. Those within heteronormativity survive, those without die. Beckett's death obviates the possibility of him being reinstated in his job which would have meant re-placing the other in the midst of its abjecting environment. The fine levied by the judge does justice to the symbolic order of the law which requires atonement for the unfair dismissal of Andrew Beckett for suffering from a debilitating disease, whilst not disturbing its embodiment, heteronormativity, in the structures of daily interaction. The senior partners can remain amongst themselves untroubled by the presence of an other who might disturb their boundaries. That other is dis-embodied through his death. This closure reinstates the order in the law firm as it was before Beckett's homosexuality was ever known. In this sense, the film affirms the line taken in the supplement to the 1973 Federal Vocational Rehabilitation Act quoted within *Philadelphia* which prohibits discrimination on the grounds of disability. This supplement states that post-1973 judgements in cases related to HIV/AIDS upheld the 1973 ruling since 'the prejudice surrounding AIDS exacts a social death which precedes the actual physical one'. *Philadelphia* complicates this position as it reveals that the social death exacted – which in Beckett's case is only partial since his family in the main rallies behind him and he finds a lawyer who, though initially reluctant, takes his case on[11] – is not one associated with HIV/AIDS but with homosexuality. The ostracism Mrs Benedict experiences does not extend to dismissal from her job. But then she is also only a paralegal adviser (thus in a much more marginal occupational position than Beckett is) and has not penetrated into the inner sanctum of legal seniority in the way that Beckett has. Moreover, as a woman she is already 'othered' and thus viewed as not exactly the same as the male senior partners. In Beckett's case this is different. His dissimulation has made him appear to be the same as the senior partners. The price exacted for this threat to the socio-professional order is therefore higher. Mrs Benedict would not have presented the same degree of threat in the first place – her femininity prevents that.

Visibility as trap

In *Unmarked* Phelan (1993) suggests that 'visibility is a trap ... it summons surveillance and the law' (6).[12] This sums up what occurs in

Philadelphia where Beckett's invisibility as a homosexual initially allows a successful professional existence through the maintenance of a separation of the private and the public, of his enactment of being gay at home from his performance of passing in public. Once his homosexuality becomes visible through the lesions on his face, his performance of passing is uncovered and the law, embodied variously in Beckett himself as a lawyer, the lawyers in Beckett's firm, the lawyer Beckett employs to defend his case, the judge and the law court in which the trial takes place, is summoned. Visibility thus becomes the trap which reveals Beckett's identity as homosexual, leads to his dismissal and a social death of kinds, and ultimately prefigures his actual, physical death.

That visibility is a function of Beckett's corporeality rather than his enactment of sexual identity. The body, in this instance, will not be denied and breaks out of its closet through the manifestation of Kaposi's sarcoma. Against the possibility of certain kinds of performance such as passing and being a competent lawyer, *Philadelphia* sets the physical reality of the infected body which confounds those performances – following his dismissal Beckett does not have to pass any more and he does not practise law again. It is, in *Philadelphia*, as if a certain 'truth' will not be denied[13] – Beckett is gay and he has to die for this, however sympathetic his character and however competent his performances may be. This is not true of his foil Mrs Benedict but then, one might argue, she was not hiding, and being of the mainstream did not have to hide, anything. Beckett's performance, justified though it may be in terms of the homophobia manifested by the senior partners which suggests that they might never have taken him on, let alone promoted him to senior associate, had they known of his homosexuality, is none the less viewed in terms of concealment and calculated disavowal within the film. It indexes the double bind he finds himself in: unlikely to make it professionally if he affirms his homosexuality, his passing makes him equally vulnerable to those around him. This is the dilemma which Phelan (1993) evades in her discussion of the problematic of visibility politics, for effectively both visibility and invisibility can constitute traps for those marginalized in mainstream society seeking representation. Beckett is made to experience this not only through his expulsion from his job when he becomes 'visible' to the senior partners but also when he looks for a lawyer to represent him in court against his former employer. He is turned down by nine other lawyers before Joe Miller, a black man,[14] agrees to take his case on, and then only in response to witnessing the extent to which Beckett is discriminated against in public.

The provisionality of performance

The film points to the temporality of performance. As it pursues the notion that 'the truth will out' (Beckett's homosexuality is revealed and so is the senior partners' homophobia), it does so by suggesting that dissonant performances will be unmasked as untrue and rebound on those who enact them. Beckett is dismissed and dies; the senior partners are fined and publicly humiliated. Within the moral economy of the film theirs is, of course, the lesser cost since their position defends the hegemony of heteronormativity – it is quite clear that they will survive their unmasking while Beckett does not. Their bodies, both as physical entities and as corporate structures, remain intact; Beckett's is obliterated.

In her analysis of the notion of performance Phelan (1993) states: 'Performance's only life is in the present. Performance cannot be saved ... Performance's being, like the ontology of subjectivity proposed here, becomes itself through disappearance' (146). Performance's life takes place at the moment of performance. It gestures towards a moment of non-performance or a moment of another performance which may be in the past or in the future. The moment of performance is thus set against the moment when the performance is not, that is is not happening or has changed into something else. Hence the idea of disappearance. Performance here is understood not in the Butlerian sense of a performative subjectivity but as a staged process the stagedness of which is explicit, and separated from other 'naturalized' and iterative performances such as the performance of everyday tasks. Phelan's notion of performance's life being tied to the present and being temporal is complexly replayed in *Philadelphia*. Importantly, some of the key performances are initiated through a process of involuntary visibilization, the visibilization of the body marked as different through KS lesions. Beckett feels forced to perform heteronormativity and health in the face of the senior partners' homophobia. He literally puts on a face when he seeks to mask the lesions with a make-up which, while it supposedly works best for hiding lesions, has a powerful and therefore revealing orange tinge. This theatricalizes Beckett's masking in the direction of clowning, and the exaggeratedness of make-up clowns wear. It thus heightens the performative quality of his pretence. Simultaneously, Beckett's body itself generates its own temporal performances, with the lesions appearing and disappearing, being more or less visible, and his health – though generally deteriorating in keeping with the film's moral economy – varying between better and worse states.

Beckett's unstable bodily performances suggest the limits of his control over his performances, and, indeed, the film reinforces the notion of performance as temporal, limited not simply by time but by factors beyond the control of the individual such as the body itself which will not be denied. Just as Beckett's performance of heteronormativity is unmasked, so is the senior partners' pretence that they fired Beckett for poor professional performance. In Beckett's case the film invokes the body as the limit of human control – Beckett is ultimately incapable of denying his illness and therefore his homosexuality beyond a certain point. Simultaneously, the partners are unmasked by the law. As the film *Philadelphia* moves towards closure, it presents a graduated or staged disappearance of its main subject reflective of its moral economy which suggests that there are 'true' selves which can be denied only for a time, that these can be discovered and dealt with accordingly. Beckett is gay; he may, temporarily, be able to perform heteronormativity but eventually his body will reveal his 'true' nature. That 'true' gay nature is incompatible with a dominant heteronormative discourse which, whilst preaching tolerance, cannot tolerate 'deviance' within its midst. It may well be, as Beckett's lawyer points out, that the trial is all about homosexuality and people's attitudes towards that, but in a liberal and supposedly tolerant country this cannot be made to be at stake. Invoking a Federal Act associated with issues of disability thus circumvents the debate about (attitudes towards) homosexuality while enabling the punishment of prejudice, deflected on to prejudice concerning disability. The debate about homosexuality is displaced and (re-)silenced through a deflection on to HIV/AIDS.

At the same time, a sanitization effect is created through the staged disappearance of the protagonist: initially fired from his job, he is also constructed as ill unto death so that his death produces the 'longed-for' closure of a film with mainstream ambitions. These ambitions mean that the film has to pander to the anxieties of those who regard homosexuality as deviant, while deflecting from the implicit intolerance of a society that prides itself on its liberalism allowing intolerance to override actual merit. Beckett's outstanding performance as a lawyer cannot save him from being punished for performing heteronormativity. His 'social', or rather 'professional' death prefigures his actual death which in itself constitutes the close of the film and confirms the heteronormative social order. Since his long-term gay partner is Spanish-speaking, thus already to some extent, even in the USA, 'other' and seemingly not HIV-positive, he does not need to be accounted for further – accepted in Beckett's family and treated well by them, he is not of the family and therefore already other. In *Philadelphia* the threat is not what is visibly other, since that can be contained, but the one who seems the same and is not.

The mirror scene

This is made evident in the mirror scene[15] which takes place in the courtroom and becomes one of the key planks of both parties' argument in the trial. The senior partners' defence team attempt to prove that the partners did not know about Beckett's lesions by suggesting that his lesions cannot be seen. To prove this their lawyer holds up a mirror to Beckett sitting in the dock, and asks whether, truthfully, he can see the lesion he has on his face from three feet away. To present Beckett's face in the mirror, the camera cuts to a position slightly to Beckett's side and from behind his left shoulder so that the viewer, whilst on the same side as Beckett, sees the mirror, side by side with the lawyer's face, at a slight angle. There is therefore no immediate identification of the viewer with Beckett – the viewer is not put in Beckett's place. Beckett, looking into the mirror, turns his head slightly to get a better look at his lesion. He cannot see it, supposedly because the mark is very faint. Neither can the viewer. The case of the invisibility of the lesion appears to be proved. In fact, a deception is practised on the viewer since Beckett has a lesion on the left side of his face but to 'find' it in the mirror he turns the right side of his face towards it. The film registers no awareness of this deception, possibly in the hope that the film audience will not notice it, possibly because the re-playing of the scene which follows heightens the dramatic impact and reinforces in an over-determined way the gradual unmasking of Beckett and the senior partners.

Beckett's own lawyer then asks if he has lesions such as the ones he had at the time of his dismissal anywhere on his body. Beckett has such lesions on his torso and is prevailed upon to reveal them. As Beckett, physically weakened by his illness, laboriously opens his shirt, the film signals the unmasking – in this instance of the senior partners' deception in pretending that they could not see his lesions. Beckett's unmasking as gay and suffering from AIDS prefigures theirs – in revealing himself, he reveals them. Holding up the mirror to Beckett again, his lawyer asks if he can see the lesions on his torso and, of course, he and the audience, both in the courtroom and the film audience, can. The camera, moving between Beckett's torso and the courtroom audience at this time, registers their horror and pity as they observe Beckett's marked body in recognition of his impending death, his otherness thus sealed.

This scene plays with notions of identity and identification. Facially Beckett looks ill but not too different from the audience. The mirror held up to him by the senior partners' lawyer is positioned off-centre and angled so that the film viewer is not placed into an identificatory space with Beckett. His semi-averted gaze into the mirror objectifies him further for the film audience whilst the simultaneous view of the lawyer (the mirror and the lawyer's face remaining side by side in this shot) keeps the notion of an audience literally in view. When his own lawyer holds the mirror up to Beckett the focus is on his torso. Beckett's face does not appear in the mirror. He has become a body, and his marked body, now revealed, makes visible his difference from the audience: he is a marked man. The horror and pity of the court room audience is that of a group of people coming face to face with the abject. Throughout this scene Beckett is objectified. As the object of everybody's gaze he is, in a sense, dehumanized – he becomes the body which betrays him as other, the body that will not be denied but the difference of which means death. 'Let's see what we're talking about', his lawyer says as he asks to see the lesions on the torso. As the film makes clear, we are talking about the highly visible, bodily marks of difference. At this point in the film the audience can 'afford' to feel not only horror but also pity since Beckett is clearly a marked man, beyond redemption, and about to die. There is no longer any threat emanating from Beckett who is so obviously near death. Even his homophobic former colleagues are moved to express distress at his sight. Through the mirror scene visible difference is thus asserted, and the imminent expulsion of the 'deviant' subject guaranteed whilst identification with that subject is contained through the camera positioning which ensures the continued viewing of Beckett as an object.

'Them' and 'us'

Philadelphia is a film troubled to the end by the notion of the 'deviant' body in our midst. This trouble is resolved through Beckett's death, required by the moral economy of mainstream representation. But, as indicated earlier, the film straddles the boundary between dying from and living with AIDS. Thus it registers the multiplicity of bodies which can suffer from AIDS through the presentation of both Beckett, and Mrs Benedict as 'blameless victim'. The latter's survival in the face of Beckett's death, however, constructs a judgement between the two characters in which she emerges as 'acceptable' and may, therefore, live while he does not and has to be killed. As Illman (1993a) puts it: 'As for dying, all those strange, marginal, "at-risk" groups can do that for us' (2). There is thus an irony in Beckett's lawyer's demand in court to bring 'it out of the closet', 'to have it out in the open' – 'it' here referring to sexual orientation. The judge may well respond that in his courtroom justice is done irrespective of colour, creed and, indeed, sexual orientation but the film belies that very assertion through its differential treatment of Mrs Benedict and Mr Beckett whose names – their alliteration suggesting the similarity of their situation – while close are not identical since their filmic fate is, indeed, not identical. *Philadelphia* makes clear that while there is a multiplicity of diverse bodies which may have HIV/AIDS, judgement is passed among these bodies, with some emerging as 'blameless' victims and others as the secretive carriers of a deadly disease which will kill them, if not others they come into contact with. At the same time, the film registers the unease of a patriarchal society which finds it difficult to reinforce the boundaries it sets up between what is and what is not acceptable. The elevation of Beckett to senior associate prior to the discovery of his illness and the recognition that he is gay reveals the impossibility of distinguishing effectively between 'them' and 'us' which the homophobic partners of the firm would like to believe in. Indeed, the social scenes which these partners are depicted in are themselves ambivalent spaces of homosociality[16] which simultaneously point to male homoerotic desire and its suppression or repression in the senior male partners.[17] At the same time the film reinforces the notion that certain kinds of visibility lead to, or reinforce, persecution and expulsion. Beckett may 'win' legally but he loses his life while the partners get away with a fine. His empowerment is thus strictly temporary, his expulsion permanent. Within the film Beckett may play a central role but that centrality is limited to a present which prefigures his disappearance and stands in inverse relation to his ultimate marginalization.

No end in sight

Philadelphia offers only two images of people with AIDS which it presents in terms of mainstream conventions. As the previous chapters have indicated, however, the emergence of HIV/AIDS led to a proliferation of images around HIV/AIDS, including those of people with and without HIV/AIDS. The history of the health promotion campaigns[18] in particular makes clear how changes in knowledge about HIV/AIDS have impacted on their representation, leading to increasing ranges of images, none of which is sufficient to capture HIV/AIDS. HIV/AIDS has thus produced an excess of meaning in line with the notion of an epidemic as an uncontainable phenomenon.

It has been suggested that HIV/AIDS may burn itself out before a cure is found. In his 1993 series on AIDS in *The Guardian* Mike Bygrave, for example, stated that 'it remains a medical rule of thumb that there are no cures for viral diseases', that, however, 'many viral infections ... [are] self-limiting' and 'that plagues and epidemics, while they come, also go' (1993: 32). Heterosexualizing the relationship between virus and host[19] Bygrave asserts: 'Unsuccessful parasites are the ones that kill their hosts and soon run into an evolutionary cul de sac themselves. Successful parasites learn to coexist with their hosts (and vice versa), settling down to a stable, long-term relationship, a biological marriage as opposed to the fatal attraction of a killer epidemic' (32). Bygrave suggests that 'evolution may take care of AIDS before we do' and that 'epidemics have come and gone without our curing them and that may be the case with AIDS too' (32). This expression of a desire for the disappearance of the disease along naturalizing lines of evolutionary progression in the face of human inability to cope with the epidemic is a way of countering the fact of the overwhelming numbers and diversity of people with HIV/AIDS (UNAIDS/WHO 1998).

Bygrave's evocation of evolution points to the desire for an HIV/AIDS history with a past and a future. This history may not be explicable but it gestures towards a bordered narrative with a beginning, a middle and an end. At present no end to the AIDS epidemic is in sight. HIV/AIDS has, in the main, in the UK vanished from public view. It has become a news item among many, an arena of abiding concern for those affected and specialists but not the 'general public' here. The proliferation of images around HIV/AIDS which characterized the period between the late 1980s and the mid-1990s has faded. We have learnt to live with HIV/AIDS in the sense that it is no longer 'new' and therefore 'noteworthy' to us. HIV/AIDS remains fraught with uncertainties but these have not affected white western heterosexual populations in ways that reduce the complacency which underlies films like *Philadelphia*. On the contrary: the image of the person with HIV/AIDS remains firmly other. Nowhere is that clearer than in the devastating figures produced by UNAIDS and the World Health Organization in their 'AIDS epidemic update' of December 1998 cited on p. 179. These global figures mask a reality which emerges in UNAIDS/WHO's textual summary of the situation: 'The epidemic has not been overcome anywhere. Virtually every country in the world has seen new infections in 1998 and the epidemic is frankly out of control in many places' (2). Significantly, 'More than 95% of all HIV-infected people now live in the developing world, which has likewise experienced 95% of all deaths to date from AIDS' (2). This concentration of HIV/AIDS in a sphere other than the white, western, heterosexual one has helped to perpetuate the othering of HIV/AIDS in western cultural consciousness. According to UNAIDS/WHO, 'in North America and Western Europe, new combinations of anti-HIV drugs continue to reduce AIDS deaths significantly' though 'the proportion of the population living with HIV has actually grown' (1998: 6). The treatments referred to here are too expensive and complicated for many of the countries most adversely affected to administer (Gwatkin 1997; Oppenheimer and Reckitt 1997: 4; Adler 1998; *Lancet* Editorial 1998; UK NGO AIDS Consortium 1998). Very significant discrepancies are thus emerging between the north and the south in terms of these hemispheres' ability to cope with HIV/AIDS. The new major divide is between the north and the south, rather than between gays and straights within northern communities. While no longer considered out of control in North America and western Europe, the epidemic has however 'not been stopped' either (UNAIDS/WHO 1998: 6). But 'HIV infections are increasingly concentrated in the poorer sectors of the population' (UNAIDS/WHO 1998: 6) whose access to cultural representation and presentation in cultural representation is, of course, much more limited than that of the (predominantly) white professional middle classes as portrayed, for instance, in *Philadelphia*. Inside that privileged circle HIV/AIDS has to be obliterated and/or disavowed, those suffering from it excluded or marginalized. Phelan (1993) suggests that 'all looking is an attempt to find a mirror' (25), a mirror which reflects the self. However, the visual field constitutes a trap since it promises to show all even though it cannot do so (Phelan 1993: 24). When Beckett looks in the mirror for the first time, he cannot see his lesion so that the mirror fails to reveal the reality of his situation, namely that he has AIDS and, indeed, Kaposi's sarcoma lesions. Only when asked about lesions elsewhere does Beckett reveal visible lesions and thus show his status as HIV-positive. The lesions do not show Beckett's homosexuality, which has however already been discussed repeatedly during the trial, in the same way that Mrs Benedict's lesions did not indicate her heterosexuality. This creates in the viewer the sense of something existing elsewhere, beyond the image both in the object beheld and in terms of what the looker desires to see – the confirmation of something the looker thinks she or he knows (already). Implicated in what is seen is thus the looker whose searching eye seeks to reveal more than the visual field will yield. In *Philadelphia* the searching eye is 'satisfied' through the revelation of the clearly visible lesions on Beckett's torso which correspond to the sense that he is a very sick man, doomed to die. The looker, if not infected by HIV and not suffering from Kaposi's sarcoma, is further satisfied that what is seen is not like her or him. Visibility thus registers as difference, the condition for separation, which is the necessary ground of maintaining the illusion of an intact self, separate from that of the gay person with HIV/AIDS, for example.

One might argue that a similar effect is generated through UNAIDS/WHO's global HIV/AIDS surveillance figures which locate HIV/AIDS firmly as existing in the main outside the western hemisphere (UNAIDS/WHO 1998: 5). Between them, *Philadelphia* and the UNAIDS/WHO figures provide one account for the decline in visibility in western cultural representation of HIV/AIDS. If the moral economy of *Philadelphia* demands the expulsion of the gay subject, achieved through his death from AIDS, then the survival of that subject, his living with HIV/AIDS, would put into question that moral economy by demanding, for example, Beckett's reinstatement into his job. The only person in that film permitted to live with HIV/AIDS is Mrs Benedict, the 'blameless victim,' whose HIV-positive status simply reinforces her position as powerless and object, already prefigured by her femininity. The film can thus 'afford' her otherness in ways in which it cannot tolerate Beckett's.

Beyond the film, though, lurks the question of those living with HIV/AIDS outside representation, in the 'real' so to speak. If part of the drive towards the proliferation of images around HIV/AIDS was an attempt at stemming the tide of infection and death, then the abatement of death from AIDS in western cultures in the second half of the 1990s (UNAIDS/WHO 1998: 6) has interrupted that flow and the images associated with it. The portrayal of people living with HIV/AIDS, often promoted by organizations seeking to help HIV-positive persons to come to terms with their condition and to re-value their lives when they seemed to be, or were assumed to be, under threat of death, raises very different issues from those related to the issue of dying from AIDS. From the viewpoint of the hegemonic discourses of western cultures they raise the question of how we relate to those whom we perceive to be different from ourselves, those who are 'othered' in our cultures. Death precludes such interrogations; living demands them. One way in which the question is answered is through silencing and invisibilizing. Now that we 'live with' HIV/AIDS, its threat seems to be diminished. Western cultural mainstream representation is unlikely to create many images of people living with HIV/AIDS since the 'other' – whatever form she or he takes – remains marginalized as part of the continual policing of the boundaries between the included and the excluded. Already in 1991 Wojnarowicz could write: 'I have attended a number of memorials in the last five years and at the last one I attended I found myself suddenly experiencing something akin to rage. I realized halfway through the event that I had witnessed a good number of the same people participating in other previous memorials. What made me angry was realizing that the memorial had little reverberation outside the room it was held in. A tv commercial for handiwipes had a higher impact on the society at large' (1991: 121–2). The experience he details of the privatization of grieving for those lost to AIDS reflects the beginnings of the invisibilization of HIV/AIDS which at present has reached heights nobody would have dreamt of ten years ago. The UNAIDS/WHO report (1998) makes clear why HIV/AIDS is viewed as happening to others and those 'othered': the bulk of the growth in infections and deaths is occurring among the most disenfranchised communities in the world,[20] those with least representation of any kind. The celebration of AIDS activism among gay men as a key tool in shifting public perceptions on HIV/AIDS in the late 1980s and early 1990s, an activism which generated responses through high visibility and visibilizing measures, has no equivalent among most of the groups and communities also powerfully affected by HIV/AIDS. The threat of spread, which temporarily mobilized heterosexual communities in the northern hemisphere, seems to have abated and encouraged renewed inertia among the populations which have perhaps the greatest power to effect change.

The reasons for this re-invisibilization of HIV/AIDS are then manifold. The recognition of the diversity of HIV/AIDS patterns across the world has led to the abandonment of the notion of a single, global epidemic. The initial, catastrophic grand narrative of HIV/AIDS has been superseded by a fragmentation and consequent proliferation of HIV/AIDS discourses which tend to engage with the specificities of particular situations and circumstances. One glance through the issues of *The Lancet* from the last four or five years makes that abundantly clear. Reports it carried on topics such as the infection of monogamous women in China who are commercial plasma donors (Wu *et al.* 1995); HIV in sub-Saharan Africa (Cooper *et al.* 1998; Gilks and Haran 1995); or the prevalence of pneumocystis carinii in Africa (Malin *et al.* 1995; Russian and Kovacs 1995) point to the fragmentation of HIV/AIDS discourses which accompany an enhanced understanding of the infection and associated illnesses. The result, not unlike the effects of the splintering of social movements into single-issue groups, has been the uneven (re)distribution of political investment in promoting change, with some groups supporting particular situations and circumstances emerging as more successful than others in attracting resources and enabling change. As Oppenheimer and Reckitt (1997) state, 'the idea of a single global epidemic is profoundly unhelpful to those who are interested in implementing prevention, treatment, and care programmes' (2) but the recognition of that diversity of needs has also led to HIV/AIDS being and continuing to be profoundly 'othered', and along health and economic lines. Phelan (1993) suggests that 'identity is perceptible only through a relation to an other – which is to say, it is a form of both resisting and claiming the other, declaring the boundary where the self diverges from and merges with the other. In that declaration of identity and identification, there is always loss, the loss of not-being the other and yet remaining dependent on that other for self-seeing, self-being' (13). But if the price of the self is the maintenance of an injured other, what careful blindness is being nurtured?

Notes

1 See also Gorna (1996: 337–77).

2 In 1985 the Lesbian and Gay Media Group felt compelled to produce a booklet to accompany a BBC2 programme entitled *A Plague On You* (broadcast at 10.25pm, 4 November 1985) in order to counter some of the misinformation which had been spread about HIV/AIDS.

3 This is evident not only in the discussions about the origins of HIV/AIDS (see Chapter 4; Chirimuurta and Chirimuurta 1987) but also, for instance, in the moves from 'heterosexualizing' AIDS to 're-gaying' it which informed the early to mid-1990s (see Oppenheimer 1997; Scott 1997).

4 See Treichler (1988b: 205–13) for an analysis of the impact of the death of Rock Hudson on public consciousness regarding HIV/AIDS.

5 In their 1998 AIDS epidemic update report UNAIDS/WHO include a section entitled 'Invisible no longer' stating that 'In industrialized countries AIDS activists succeeded in raising the profile of the epidemic early on. But in the developing world where most men and women with HIV live, it is only now, two decades after the virus first started spreading, that the repercussions of AIDS are stripping off its cloak of invisibility' (7). This geographical displacement of AIDS is one of the contributing factors in the (re)invisibilization of AIDS.

6 Oppenheimer and Reckitt's (1997) volume is in part intended to counteract this notion.

7 Beckett's assumed heterosexuality is underscored by his close family ties and his interest in familial matters such as his asking after the newly born daughter of the lawyer he employs to fight his case against the law firm for him. Significantly, the film focuses predominantly on his relations and positions within various heterosexually invested arenas.

8 For the construction of women in relation to HIV/AIDS within mainstream conventions see Gorna (1996); Roth and Fuller (1998); Roth and Hogan (1998); Richardson (1987). For a rather more problematic gendered view of AIDS see Foreman 1999.

9 This is, of course, not inevitably the case but is constructed as such within this film.

10 Whilst Kaposi's sarcoma is 'a common manifestation of AIDS in men ... women rarely develop KS' (Bury 1994: 36). When they do so it can be because of a blood transfusion or if they have acquired HIV heterosexually, through a bisexual partner. *Philadelphia* draws on this situation.

11 It has to be noted that Beckett's lawyer is black and working on his own rather than in a prestigious law firm – an index of the prejudices of which he is object, but also of his independence and the notion of the importance of alliances among those discriminated against as a means of getting justice.

12 Phelan (1993) questions the efficacy of the visibility politics which she thinks have dominated the 1980s and early 1990s. She doubts that 'greater visibility of the hitherto under-represented leads to enhanced political power' (2). ACT UP's work, discussed in Chapter 2, contradicts Phelan's viewpoint. For a discussion of the impact of visibility politics on the political process see Aronowitz (1995).

13 This conforms to the realist conventions which underpin this film.

14 The video cover for *Philadelphia* says of Miller that 'although he has grown up knowing the pain of prejudice, he's never before had to confront his own prejudices against homosexuality and AIDS ... until now.' Experiencing marginalization similar to that of Beckett does not necessarily, as the film reveals, promote alliances among those discriminated against.

15 Such mirror scenes feature commonly in film dealing with HIV/AIDS, representing both the searching for symptoms of the disease and the moment of recognition of that disease when – usually – KS lesions are found. The use of the mirror as an emblem of identity and its destabilization through the simultaneous being and not-being in materiality has a long cultural history. Abrams (1953) produced a classic text on the subject in relation to romantic theory.

16 In using the term 'homosociality' I refer to Eve Kosofsky Sedgwick's (1985) discussion of depictions of homosociality in nineteenth-century literature and her definition of the term: '"Homosocial" is a word occasionally used in history and the social sciences, where it describes social bonds between persons of the same sex; it is a neologism, obviously formed by analogy with "homosexual," and just as obviously meant to be distinguished from "homosexual." In fact, it is applied to such activities as "male bonding," which may, as in our society, be characterized by intense homophobia, fear and hatred of homosexuality' (1).

17 Butler (1997) produces an extended pertinent argument (chapter 5) about the establishment of gender 'by a set of disavowed attachments' (147). She suggests that 'a masculine gender is formed from the refusal to grieve the masculine as a possibility of love' (146) which leads to heterosexual melancholy.

18 A summary of these can be found in Field, Wellings and McVey 1997: 87–93.

19 For a discussion of the genderization of science through the use of gendered descriptions and metaphors see Martin (1991).

20 Foreman's (1999) *AIDS and Men* utilizes as chapter headings for Part 2, the largest section of the book, place names: 'Mexico, Tanzania, Ghana, Uganda, Kenya, Russia, Brazil, Malawi, Thailand, Ivory Coast, Bangladesh'. Here we have the 'others' referred to in the text prominently on display.

References

Abrams, M. H. (1953), *The Mirror and the Lamp: Romantic Theory and the Critical Tradition*, Oxford, Oxford University Press.

Abu-Lughod, J. (1989), On the remaking of history; how to reinvent the past, in B. Kruger and P. Mariani (eds), *Remaking History*, Seattle, Bay Press, 1989.

ACT-UP/New York Women and AIDS Book Group (1990), *Women, AIDS and Activism*, Boston, MA, South End Press.

Adams, M. L. (1988), All that rubber, all that talk, in I. Rieder and P. Ruppelt (eds), *Matters of Life and Death: Women Speak About AIDS*, Pittsburgh, Cleis Press, 1988; rpt London, Virago, 1989.

Adams, P. (1996), *The Emptiness of the Image*, London, Routledge.

Adler, M. W. (1998), Antiretrovirals in the developing world, *The Lancet*, 351, 24 January, 232.

Ahmed, S. (1998), Animated borders: skin, colour and tanning, in M. Shildrick and J. Price (eds), *Vital Signs: Feminist Reconfigurations of the Bio/logical Body*, Edinburgh, Edinburgh University Press.

AID-CH (ed.) (n.d.), Information on Anti-AIDS poster campaigns from around the world, Zurich, Medienstelle Verleih BILD + TON.

Aids-snub nurse dropped (1990), *The Guardian*, 15 December, Home Page, 2.

Aldridge, D. (1990), Waiting to be loved, *The Guardian*, 1 March, Features, 36.

Altman, D. (1994), Psycho-cultural responses to AIDS, in T. Gott (ed.), *Don't Leave Me This Way: Art in the Age of AIDS*, Melbourne, Thames and Hudson, 1994.

Aronowitz, S. (1995), Against the liberal state: ACT-UP and the emergence of postmodern politics, in L. Nicholson and S. Seidman (eds), *Social Postmodernism: Beyond Identity Politics*, Cambridge, Cambridge University Press, 1995.

Artenstein, A. W., Coppola, J., Brown, A. E. *et al.* (1995), Multiple introductions of HIV-1 subtype E into the western hemisphere, *The Lancet*, 346, 4 November, 1197–8.

Atkins, R. (1989), Photographing AIDS, in J. Z. Grover (ed.), *AIDS: The Artists' Response*, Columbus, Hoyt L. Sherman Gallery.

Bailey, A. S. and G. Corbitt (1996), Was HIV present in 1959?, Letter to the editor, *The Lancet*, 347, 20 January, 189.

Bannon, A. (1959), *I Am a Woman*, rpt Tallahasse, Naiad Press, 1986.

Barthes, R. (1986a), *The Rustle of Language*, trans. Farrar, Straus, and Giroux, Inc., Oxford, Basil Blackwell.

Barthes, R. (1986b), The death of the author, in *The Rustle of Language*, trans. Farrar, Straus and Giroux, Inc., Oxford, Basil Blackwell, 1986.

Barthes, R. (1986c), The reality effect, in *The Rustle of Language*, trans. Farrar, Straus and Giroux, Inc., Oxford, Basil Blackwell, 1986.

Barthes, R. (1977; rpt 1982), *Image Music Text*, London, Fontana.

Barthes, R. (1973), *S/Z*, trans. Farrar, Straus and Giroux, Inc., Oxford, Blackwell, 1990.

Beer, G. (1996), 'Authentic tidings of invisible things': vision and the invisible in the later nineteenth century, in T. Brennan and M. Jay (eds), *Vision in Context: Historical and Contemporary Perspectives on Sight*, London, Routledge.

Bhatt, C. and R. Lee (1997), Official knowledges: the free market, identity formation, sexuality and race in the HIV/AIDS sector, in J. Oppenheimer and H. Reckitt (eds), *Acting on AIDS: Sex, Drugs and Politics*, London, Serpent's Tail.

Birke, L. (1999), *Feminism and the Biological Body*, Edinburgh, Edinburgh University Press.

Blackman, I. (1995), White girls are easy, black girls are studs, in L. Pearce and J. Stacey (eds), *Romance Revisited*, London, Lawrence and Wishart.

Blake, N., Rinder, L., and A. Scholder (eds) (1995), *In a Different Light: Visual Culture, Sexual Identity, Queer Practice*, San Francisco, City Lights Books.

Blue (1993), dir. D. Jarman, FaxVideo.

Boffin, T. (1990a), Angelic rebels: lesbians and safer sex, in T. Boffin and S. Gupta (eds), *Ecstatic Antibodies: Resisting the AIDS Mythology*, London, Rivers Oram Press.

Boffin, T. (1990b), Fairy tales, 'facts', and gossip: lesbians and AIDS, in T. Boffin and S. Gupta (eds), *Ecstatic Antibodies: Resisting the AIDS Mythology*, London, Rivers Oram Press.

Boffin, T. (1989), Artist's statement, in J. Z. Grover (ed.), *AIDS: The Artists' Response*, Columbus, Hoyt L. Sherman Gallery.

Boffin, T. and J. Fraser (eds) (1991), *Stolen Glances: Lesbians Take Photographs*, London, Pandora.

Boffin, T. and S. Gupta (eds) (1990), *Ecstatic Antibodies: Resisting the AIDS Mythology*, London, Rivers Oram Press.

Bordo, S. (1993), *Unbearable Weight: Feminism, Western Culture and the Body*, Berkeley, California University Press.

Brabazon, T. (1993), At your own risk; Derek Jarman and the (semiotic) death of a film maker, *Social Semiotics*, 3/2, 183–200.

Bradley, R. (1992), Politicized performances: a symposium – the abnormal affair of *The Normal Heart*, *Text and Performance Quarterley*, 12, 362–71.

Braidotti, R. (1991), *Patterns of Dissonance*, Cambridge, Polity Press.

Bremner, C. (1992), Cast out for an Aids heresy, *The Times on CDRom*, 11 May, LT, 4.

Brindle, D. (1990), Aids virus carrier 'abused youths', *The Guardian*, 7 September, Home Page, 24.

Brodine, S. K., Mascola, J. R., Weiss, P. J. *et al.* (1995), Detection of diverse HIV-1 genetic subtypes in the USA, *The Lancet*, 346, 4 November, 1198–9.

Bronfen, E. (1992), *Over Her Dead Body: Death, Femininity and the Aesthetic*, Manchester, Manchester University Press.

Bronski, M. (1997), Why gay men still have unsafe sex: beauty, self-esteem and the myth of HIV-negativity, in J. Oppenheimer and H. Reckitt (eds), *Acting on AIDS: Sex, Drugs and Politics*, London, Serpent's Tail.

Bronski, M. (1989), Death and the erotic imagination, in E. Carter and S. Watney (eds), *Taking Liberties: AIDS and Cultural Politics*, London, Serpent's Tail.

Brown, J. (1992), Sex, lies and penetration: a butch finally 'fesses up', in J. Nestle (ed.), *The Persistent Desire: A Butch–Femme Reader*, Boston, Alyson Publications Inc.

Bunting, M. (1993a), Paper hits back at Aids critics, *The Guardian*, 11 December, Home Page, 3.

Bunting, M. (1993b), War of words over Aids, *The Guardian*, 13 December, G2T, 16.

Bury, J. (1994), Women and HIV/AIDS: Medical issues, in L. Doyal, J. Naidoo and T. Wilton (eds), *AIDS: Setting a Feminist Agenda*, London, Taylor & Francis.

Bury, J., Morrison, V. and S. McLachlan (eds) (1992), *Working with Women and AIDS*, London, Routledge.

Butler, B. (1990), *Ceremonies of the Heart: Celebrating Lesbian Unions*, Washington, Seal Press.

Butler, J. (1997), *The Psychic Life of Power: Theories in Subjection*, Stanford, Stanford University Press.

Butler, J. (1993), *Bodies that Matter*, London, Routledge.

Butler, J. (1992), Sexual inversions, in D. C. Stanton (ed.), *Discourses on Sexuality*, Ann Arbor, University of Michigan Press.

Butler, J. (1990), *Gender Trouble*, London, Routledge.

Bygrave, M. (1993), The story of AIDS: part three – time's enemy, *The Guardian*, 3 July, Weekend, 32.

Califia, P. (1993), *Melting Pot*, Boston, Alyson Publications, Inc.

Califia, P. (1988a), *Macho Sluts*, Boston, Alyson Press.

Califia, P. (1988b), The surprise party, in *Macho Sluts*, Boston, Alyson Press.

Callow, S. (1993), In times of plague and pestilence, *The Observer*, 26 September.

Cameron, D. (1995), Extended sensibilities: homosexual presence in contemporary art, in N. Blake, L. Rinder, and A. Scholder (eds), *In a Different Light: Visual Culture, Sexual Identity, Queer Practice*, San Francisco, City Lights Books.

Cameron, D. and E. Frazer (1987), *The Lust to Kill: A Feminist Investigation of Sexual Murder*, New York, New York University Press.

Cantacuzino, M. (1993), *Till Break of Day: Meeting the Challenge of HIV and AIDS at London Lighthouse*, London, Heinemann.

Carter, E. (1989), AIDS and critical practice, in E. Carter and S. Watney (eds), *Taking Liberties: AIDS and Cultural Politics*, London, Serpent's Tail.

Carter, E. and S. Watney (eds) (1989), *Taking Liberties: AIDS and Cultural Politics*, London, Serpent's Tail.

Cartland, B. (1987), *A Circus for Love*, London, Pan Books.

Cheim, J., Cortez, D., Gimenez, C. and K. Kertess (1993), *Drawing the Line Against AIDS*, New York, The American Foundation for AIDS Research.

Chelala, C. (1992), HIV case shocks USA, *The Lancet*, 350, 8 November, 1376.

Chirimuuta, R. C. and R. J. Chirimuuta (1987), *Aids, Africa and Racism*, Derbyshire, R. Chirimuuta.

Clum, J. M. (1992), AIDS drama: displacing *Camille*, in *Acting Gay*, New York, Columbia University Press, 1992.

Code, L. (1995), *Rhetorical Spaces: Essays on Gendered Locations*, London, Routledge.

Coles, J. (1990), HIV man jailed in sex case, *The Guardian*, 8 September, Home Page, 2.

Colvin, M., Abdool Karim, S. S. and D. Wilkinson (1995), Migration and AIDS, *The Lancet*, 346, 11 November, 1303–4.

Cooper, R. S., Rotimi, C., Kaufman, J. and T. Lawoyin (1998), Mortality data for sub-Saharan Africa, *The Lancet*, 351, 6 June, 1739–40.

Corbitt, G, Bailey, A. S. and G. Williams (1990), HIV infection in Manchester, 1959, *The Lancet*, 336, 51.

Core, P. (1989), Unseen enemy, *The Independent* 14 April, 18.

Crimp, D. (1997), Interview: Douglas Crimp in conversation with Mary Kelly, in M. Iversen, D. Crimp, and H. K. Bhabha (eds), *Mary Kelly*, London, Phaidon Press, 1997.

Crimp, D. (1993), *On the Museum's Ruins*, Cambridge, MA, MIT Press, 1995.

Crimp, D. (ed.) (1991), *AIDS: Cultural Analysis Cultural Activism*, Cambridge, MA, MIT Press.

Crimp, D. (1989a), Art and activism: a conversation between Douglas Crimp and Greg Bordowitz, in J. Z. Grover (ed.), *AIDS: The Artists' Response*, Columbus, Hoyt L. Sherman Gallery.

Crimp, D. (1989b), Mourning and militancy, *October*, 51 (winter), 3–18.

Crimp, D. and A. Rolston (1990), *AIDSdemographics*, Seattle, Bay Press.

De Beauvoir, S. (1949; rpt 1972), *The Second Sex*, Harmondsworth, Penguin.

De Certeau, M. (1997), *The Capture of Speech and Other Political Writings*, Minneapolis, University of Minnesota Press.

Decosas, J., Kane, F., Anarfi, J. K. *et al.* (1995), Migration and AIDS, *The Lancet*, 346, 23 September, 826–8.

DeHardt, D.C. (1993), Feminist therapy with heterosexual couples: the ultimate issue is domination, in S. Wilkinson and C. Kitzinger (eds), *Heterosexuality: A Feminism and Psychology Reader*, London, Sage, 1993.

Derek Jarman's Garden, 1995, London, Thames and Hudson.

Diamond, E. (1997), *Unmaking Mimesis*, London, Routledge.

Dorn, N., Henderson, S. and N. South (eds) (1992), *AIDS: Women, Drugs and Social Care*, London, Falmer Press.

Douglas, M. (1966), *Purity and Danger: An Analysis of the Concepts of Pollution and Taboo*, London, Routledge, 1995.

Doyal, L., Naidoo, J. and T. Wilton (eds) (1994), *AIDS: Setting a Feminist Agenda*, London, Taylor and Francis.

Dubin, S. C. (1992), AIDS: bearing witness, in S. C. Dubin (ed.), *Arresting Images: Impolitic Art and Uncivil Actions*, London, Routledge, 1992.

DuCille, A. (1996), *Skin Trade*, Cambridge, MA, Harvard University Press.

Duncan, N. (ed.) (1996), *Bodyspace*, London, Routledge.

Duncombe, J. and D. Marsden (1995), 'Can men love?': 'reading', 'staging' and 'resisting' the romance, in L. Pearce and J. Stacey (eds), *Romance Revisited*, London, Lawrence and Wishart.

Edelman, L. (1993), The mirror and the tank: 'AIDS,' subjectivity, and the rhetoric of activism, in T. F. Murphy and S. Poirier (eds), *Writing AIDS*, New York, Columbia University Press.

Epstein, J. (1992) AIDS, stigma, and narratives of containment, *American Imago: Studies in Psychoanalysis and Culture*, 49/3 (1992), 293–310.

Fee, E. and D. M. Fox (eds) (1988), *AIDS: The Burdens of History*, Berkeley, University of California Press.

Field, B., Wellings, K. and D. McVey (1997), *Promoting Safer Sex: The HEA's Mass Media Campaigns 1987–1996*, London, Health Education Authority.

Fineman, M. (1990), India losing its battle with Aids, *The Guardian*, 29 May, 10.

Fishman, R. H. B. (1996), Prevalence of HIV infection among Israel's Ethiopian immigrants, *The Lancet*, 347, 10 February, 389.

Fitzsimons, D., Hardy, V. and K. Tolley (eds) (1995), *The Economic and Social Impact of AIDS in Europe*, London, Cassell.

Foreman, M. (ed.) (1999), *AIDS and Men: Taking Risks or Taking Responsibility?*, London, Panos/Zed.

Foster, H. (1985), *Recodings: Art, Spectacle, Cultural Politics*, Seattle, Bay Press.

Fowler, B. (1991), *The Alienated Reader: Women and Popular Romantic Literature in the Twentieth Century*. Hemel Hempstead, Harvester Wheatsheaf.

Freud, S. (1917), Mourning and melancholia, in *On Metapsychology*, Pelican Freud Library vol. 11, Harmondsworth, Penguin, 1987.

Freud, S. (1914), On narcissism: an introduction, in *On Metapsychology*, Pelican Freud Library vol. 11, Harmondsworth, Penguin, 1987.

Frost, B. and N. Watt (1990), Changing face of life in Britain, *The Times on CDRom*, 5 December, n.p.

Frye, M. (1992), Willful virgin *or* do you have to be a lesbian to be a feminist?, in *Willful Virgin*, Freedom, CA, Crossing Press.

Frye, M. (1991), Lesbian sex, in J. Barrington (ed.), *An Intimate Wilderness: Lesbian Writers on Sexuality*, Portland, Eighth Mountain Press.

Frye, N. (1973), *Anatomy of Criticism: Four Essays*, Princeton, Princeton University Press.

Gagnon, M. (1986), Texta scientiae (the enlacing of knowledge) Mary Kelly's 'Corpus', *C Magazine*, 10, 24.

Galai, N., Kalinkovich, A., Burstein, R. *et al.* (1997), African HIV-1 subtype C and rate of progression among Ethiopian immigrants in Israel, *The Lancet*, 349, 18 January, 180–1.

Garfield, S. (1994), *The End of Innocence: Britain in the Time of AIDS*, London, Faber and Faber.

Gever, M. (1991), Pictures of sickness: Stuart Marshall's *Bright Eyes*, in D. Crimp (ed.), *AIDS: Cultural Analysis Cultural Activism*, Cambridge, MA, MIT Press, 1991.

Gilks, C. F. and D. Haran (1995), Impact of HIV in sub-Saharan Africa, *The Lancet*, 346, 15 July, 187.

Gilman, S. (1997), AIDS and stigma, in J. Oppenheimer and H. Reckitt (eds), *Acting on AIDS: Sex, Drugs and Politics*, London, Serpent's Tail.

Gilman, S. L. (1988a), *Disease and Representation: Images of Illness from Madness to AIDS*, Ithaca, Cornell University Press.

Gilman, S. L. (1988b), AIDS and syphilis: the iconography of disease, in D. Crimp (ed.), *AIDS: Cultural Analysis, Cultural Activism*, Cambridge, MA, MIT Press, 1991.

Goorney, H. and E. MacColl (eds) (1986), *Agit-prop to Theatre Workshop*, Manchester, Manchester University Press.

Gorna, R. (1997), Dangerous vessels: feminism and the AIDS crisis, in J. Oppenheimer and H. Reckitt (eds), *Acting on AIDS: Sex, Drugs and Politics*, London, Serpent's Tail.

Gorna, R. (1996), *Vamps, Virgins and Victims: How Can Women Fight AIDS?*, London, Cassell.

Gott, T. (ed.) (1994), *Don't Leave Me This Way: Art in the Age of AIDS*, Melbourne, Thames & Hudson.

Graham, S. M., Daley, H. M. and B. Ngwira (1997), Finger clubbing and HIV infection in Malawian children, *The Lancet*, 349, 4 January, 31.

Greenstreet, B. (1995), The questionnaire: Larry Kramer, *The Guardian*, 26 August, 46.

Greyson, J. (1993), *Zero Patience*, Telefilm Canada, Zero Patience Production.

Greyson, J. (1989), Parma violets for wayland flowers, in J. Z. Grover (ed.), *AIDS: The Artists' Response*, Columbus, Hoyt L. Sherman Gallery.

Griffin, G. (1997), In/corporation: Jackie Kay's *The Adoption Papers*, in V. Bertram (ed.), *Kicking Daffodils: Twentieth-century Women Poets*, Edinburgh, Edinburgh University Press.

Griffin, G. (1996), *Feminist Activism in the 1990s*, London, Taylor & Francis.

Griffin, G. (1995), Safe and sexy: lesbian erotica in the age of AIDS, in L. Pearce and J. Stacey (eds), *Romance Revisited*, London, Lawrence and Wishart, 1995.

Griffin, G. (1993), *Heavenly Love? Lesbian Images in Twentieth-Century Women's Writing*, Manchester, Manchester University Press.

Grimshaw, J. (1989), The individual challenge, in E. Carter and S. Watney (eds), *Taking Liberties: AIDS and Cultural Politics*, London, Serpent's Tail.

Gross, G. D. (1992), Coming up for air: three AIDS plays, *Journal of American Culture*, 15/2, 63–7.

Grosz, E. (1995), *Space, Time and Perversion*, London, Routledge.

Grosz, E. (1994), *Volatile Bodies: Towards a Corporeal Feminism*, Bloomington, Indiana University Press.

Grosz, E. and E. Probyn (eds) (1995), *Sexy Bodies*, London, Routledge.

Grove, V. (1990), Lone mother fighting for a singular legitimacy, *Sunday Times on CDRom*, 21 January, n.p.

Grover, J. Z. (1991), AIDS: key words, in D. Crimp (ed.), *AIDS: Cultural Analysis Cultural Activism*, Cambridge, MA, MIT Press, 1991.

Grover, J. Z. (1989a), *AIDS: The Artists' Response*, Columbus, Hoyt L. Sherman Gallery.

Grover, J. Z. (1989b), Visible lesions: images of the PWA, *Afterimage* (summer), 10–16.

Gwatkin, D. R. (1997), Global burden of disease, *The Lancet*, 350, 12 July, 141.

Haeberle, E. J. (1989), Swastika, pink triangle, and yellow star: the destruction of sexology and the persecution of homosexuals in Nazi Germany, in M. B. Duberman, M. Vicinus and G. Chauncey (eds), *Hidden From History: Reclaiming the Gay and Lesbian Past*, Harmondsworth, Penguin, 1991.

Hancock, C. (1993), Letter: The awful consequences of unlimited sex, *The Guardian*, 3 December, Features, 25.

Haraway, D. (1997), The persistence of vision, in K. Conboy, N. Medina and S. Stanbuck (eds), *Writing on the Body: Female Embodiment and Feminist Theory*, New York, Columbia University Press.

Haraway, D. (1991), *Simians, Cyborgs and Women: The Reinvention of Nature*, London, Free Association Press.

Harding, S. (1998), *Is Science Multi-cultural?* Bloomington, Indiana University Press.

Hawkins, R. and D. Cooper (1995), Against nature: a group work show of work by homosexual men, in N. Blake, L. Rinder and A. Scholder (eds), *In a Different Light: Visual Culture, Sexual Identity, Queer Practice*, San Francisco, City Lights Books.

Healey, E. and A. Mason (eds) (1994), *Stonewall 25: The Making of the Lesbian and Gay Community in Britain*, London, Virago.

Henderson, M. (1990), Shadow of fear over adoption, *The Guardian*, 12 December, Features, 23.

HIV 'vampires wreak revenge', *The Guardian*, 15 July 1993, 11.

HIV link confirmed (1995), *Times Higher Educational Supplement*, 15 September. UK news section. Version 31 July 1999. <http://www.thesis.co.uk>

Hoagland, S. L. (1988), *Lesbian Ethics: Towards New Value*, Palo Alto, Institute of Lesbian Studies.

Hogan, K. (1997), Where experience and representation collide: lesbians, feminists and the AIDS crisis, in D. Heller (ed.), *Cross-purposes: Lesbians, Feminists, and the Limits of Alliance*, Bloomington, Indiana University Press.

Holland, J., Ramazanoglu, C., Sharpe, S. and R. Thomson (1996), Pressured pleasure: young women and the negotiation of sexual boundaries, in S. Jackson and S. Scott (eds), *Feminism and Sexuality: A Reader*, Edinburgh, Edinburgh University Press.

Holland, J., Ramazanoglu, C., Scott, S. and R. Thomson (1994a), Desire, risk and control: the body as a site of contestation, in L. Doyal, J. Naidoo and T. Wilton (eds), *AIDS: Setting a Feminist Agenda*, London, Taylor & Francis.

Holland, J., Ramazanoglu, C., Sharpe, S. and R. Thomson (1994b), Achieving masculine sexuality: young men's strategies for managing vulnerability, in L. Doyal, J. Naidoo and T. Wilton (eds), *AIDS: Setting a Feminist Agenda*, London, Taylor & Francis.

Holland, J., Ramazanoglu, C., Sharpe, S. and R. Thomson, (1992), *Pressured Pleasure: Young Women and the Negotiation of Sexual Boundaries*, London, Tufnell Press.

Hollibaugh, A. (1998), Transmission, transmission, where's the transmission?, in N. L. Roth and K. Hogan (eds), *Gendered Epidemic: Representations of Women in the Age of AIDS*, London, Routledge.

Holsclaw, D. (1989) AIDS on stage, in J. Z. Grover (ed.), *AIDS: The Artists' Response*, Columbus, Hoyt L. Sherman Gallery.

Hood, C. L. (1998), Scarlett begat Kim: a counter-biography, in N. L. Roth and K. Hogan (eds), *Gendered Epidemic: Representations of Women in the Age of AIDS*, London, Routledge.

Hope, T. (1997), Melancholic modernity: the hom(m)osexual symptom and the homosocial corpse, in E. Weed and N. Schor (eds), *Feminism Meets Queer Theory*, Bloomington, Indiana University Press.

Horton, R. (1998), The 12th world AIDS conference: a cautionary tale, *The Lancet*, 352, 11 July, 122.

Howard, D. (1999), Don't throw away the condoms yet!, ACT UP Golden Gate, Archived ACT UP/Golden Gate Articles. Version 7 October 1999. <http://www.actupgg.org/BARarchive.html>

Illman, J. (1993a), Life, love and death, *The Guardian*, 30 November, G2T, 2.

Illman, J. (1993b), World aids: the carnal cabaret, *The Guardian*, 30 November, G2T, 6.

Iversen, M., Crimp, D. and H. Bhabha (eds) (1997), *Mary Kelly*, London, Phaidon Press.

Jackson, S. (1995), Women and heterosexual love: complicity, resistance and change, in L. Pearce and J. Stacey (eds), *Romance Revisited*, London, Lawrence and Wishart,.

Jacques, M. (1990), Family in a state of flux, *The Times on CDRom*, 27 June, n.p.

Jarman, D. (1994) *Chroma: A Book of Colour – June '93*, London, Century.

Jarman, D. (1993a), *Blue: Das Buch zum Film*, Berlin, Verlag Martin Schmitz.

Jarman, D. (1993b), *Queer*, London, Richard Salmon Ltd.

Jarman, D. (1993c), *Blue*, London, Artificial Eye.

Jarman, D. (n.d.), *Evil Queen*, Manchester, Whitworth Art Gallery.

Jarman, D. (1992; rpt 1993), *At Your Own Risk: A Saint's Testament*, London, Vintage.

Jarman, D. (1991; rpt 1992), *Modern Nature: The Journals of Derek Jarman*, London, Vintage.

Jeffreys, S. (1990), *Anticlimax: A Feminist Perspective on the Sexual Revolution*, London, Women's Press.

Jenkins, C. (ed.) (1995), *Visual Culture*, London, Routledge.

Jongh, N. de (1990), Media blamed for Aids hysteria, *The Guardian*, 23 August, Home Page, 7.

Juhasz, A. (1995), *AIDS TV: Identity, Community, and Alternative Video*, Durham, Duke University Press.

Kaplan, E. H. (1998), Israel's ban on use of Ethiopians' blood: how many infectious donations were prevented?, *The Lancet*, 351, 11 April, 1127–8.

Kay, J. (1998), *Off Colour*, Newcastle upon Tyne, Bloodaxe Books.

Kay, J. (1993), *Other Lovers*, Newcastle upon Tyne, Bloodaxe Books.

Kay, J. (1991), *The Adoption Papers*, Newcastle upon Tyne, Bloodaxe Books.

Keane, J. (1993), AIDS, identity and the space of desire, *Textual Practice*, 7, 453–70.

Kemp, B. (1999), She said, she said, *Diva*, September, 14–18.

Kigotho, A. W. (1997), Moi scuppers sex-education plans in Kenya, *The Lancet*, 350, 18 October, 1152.

Kimmelman, M. (1989), Bitter harvest: AIDS and the arts, *The New York Times*, 19 March, 1, 6.

King, E. (1990), AIDS to understanding, *City Limits*, 29 November–6 December 1990.

Kinsella, J. (1989), *Covering the Plague: AIDS and the American Media*, New Brunswick, Rutgers University Press.

Kitzinger, J. (1994), Visible and invisible women in AIDS discourses, in L. Doyal, J. Naidoo and T. Wilton (eds), *AIDS: Setting a Feminist Agenda*, London, Taylor & Francis.

Knutson, D. (1996), Understanding Kaposi's Sarcoma (KS), ACT UP Golden Gate, Archived ACT UP/Golden Gate Articles. Version 7 October 1999. <http://www.actupgg.org./BARarchive.html>

Kramer, L. (1994) *Reports from the Holocaust: The Story of an AIDS Activist*, London, Cassell.

Kramer, L. (1993), *The Destiny of Me*, London, Nick Hern Books.

Kramer, L. (1987), *The Normal Heart*, London, Nick Hern Books.

Kramer, L. (1983a), 1,112 and counting, in L. Kramer, *Reports from the Holocaust*, London, Cassell, 1994.

Kramer, L. (1983b), 2,339 and counting, in L. Kramer, *Reports from the Holocaust*, London, Cassell, 1994.

Krauss, R. (1990), A note on photography and the simulacral, in C. Squiers (ed.), *The Critical Image: Essays on Contemporary Photography*, Seattle, Bay Press.

Kristeva, J. (1982), *Powers of Horror: An Essay on Abjection*, trans. Leon S. Roudiez, New York, Columbia University Press.

Kruger, B. (1994), *Remote Control: Power, Cultures, and the World of Appearances*, Cambridge, MA, MIT Press.

Lancet Editorial (1998), AIDS, the unbridgable gap, *The Lancet*, 351, 20 June, 1825.

Langford, W. (1995), 'Snuglet puglet loves to snuggle with snuglet piglet': alter personalities in heterosexual love relationships, in L. Pearce and J. Stacey (eds), *Romance Revisited*, London, Lawrence and Wishart.

Lauritsen, J. (1993), Looking back on Berlin, *Rethinking AIDS Home Page*. Version 27 July 1999. <http://www.duesberg.com/jlberlin.html>

Lean, G. (1999), AIDS is world's number one killer infection, *The Independent on Sunday*, 23 May, 5.

Leonard, Z. (1990), Lesbians in the AIDS crisis, in ACT-UP/New York Women and AIDS Book Group, *Women, AIDS and Activism*, Boston, MA, South End Press.

Leroy, V., Ntawiniga, P., Nziyumvira, A. *et al.* (1995), HIV prevalence among pregnant women in Kigali, Rwanda, *The Lancet*, 346, 2 December, 1488–9.

Lesbian and Gay Media Group (1985), *'A Plague on You': AIDS, the Media and the Truth*, London, Terrence Higgins Trust.

Lorde, A. (1984), The master's tools will never dismantle the master's house, in *Sister Outsider*, Trumanburg, New York, The Crossing Press.

Lorde, A. (1980), Uses of the erotic, in L. Lederer (ed.), *Take Back the Night: Women and Pornography*, New York, William Morrow and Co.

Lupton, D. (1994), *Moral Threats and Dangerous Desires: AIDS in the News Media*, London, Taylor and Francis.

Lynch, M. (1982), Living with Kaposi's, *Body Politic*, 88, November, 31-7.

Malin, A. S., Gwanzura, L. K. Z., Klein, S. *et al.* (1995), *Pneumocystis carinii* in Zimbabwe, *The Lancet*, 346, 11 November, 1258.

Mann, G. (1999), The Scrimshaw butch, in T. Taormino (ed.), *Best Lesbian Erotica 1999*, San Francisco, Cleis Press.

Manning, O. (1974; rpt 1983), *The Rainforest*, Harmondsworth, Penguin.

Marshall, S. (1990), Picturing deviancy, in T. Boffin and S. Gupta (eds), *Ecstatic Antibodies: Resisting the AIDS Mythology*, London, Rivers Oram Press.

Martin, E. (1991), The egg and the sperm: how science has constructed a romance based on stereotypical male-female roles, *Signs: Journal of Women in Culture and Society*, 16/31, 485–501.

Martin, E. (1987), *The Woman in the Body*, Buckingham, Open University Press.

Mason-John, V. (1991), Pride of place: Valerie Mason-John profiles Jackie Kay, one of Britain's most promising young poets, *The Guardian*, 10 October, Features, 38.

Mayes, S. and L. Stein (eds) (1993), *Positive Lives: Responses to HIV – A Photodocumentary*, London, Cassell.

McGregor, A. (1983), WHO says AIDS no risk to the public at large, *The Times*, 29 October.

McKie, R. and O. Timbs (1984), Why AIDS battle is being lost, *The Observer*, 25 November.

McMillan, C. (1982), *Women, Reason and Nature*, Oxford, Basil Blackwell.

Merck, M. (1993), A case of AIDS, in *Perversions*, London, Virago.

Meyer, R. (1995), This is to enrage you: Gran Fury and the graphics of AIDS activism, in N. Felshin (ed.), *But What Is Art? The Spirit of Art as Activism*, Seattle, Bay Press.

Mihill, C. (1990a), Minister backs adoption by race, *The Guardian*, 30 January, Home Page, 2.

Mihill, C. (1990b), Manchester man had HIV 31 years ago, *The Guardian*, 6 July, Home page, 24.

Miller, D. A. (1993), Sontag's urbanity, in N. Blake, L. Rinder and A. Scholder (eds), *In a Different Light: Visual Culture, Sexual Identity, Queer Practice*, San Francisco, City Lights Books.

Miller, D. and K. Williams (1993), Negotiating HIV/AIDS information: agendas, media strategies and the news, in J. Eldrigge (ed.), *Getting the Message: News, Truth and Power*, London, Routledge.

Miller, N. and R. C. Rockwell (eds) (1988), *AIDS in Africa: The Social and Policy Implications*, Lewiston, Edwin Mellen Press, and Washington, The National Council for International Health.

Mitchell, P. (1992), Cypriot sentenced for infecting woman with HIV-1, *The Lancet*, 350, 9 August, 422.

Morgan, S. (1996), Borrowed time, in R. Wollen (ed.), *Derek Jarman: A Portrait*, London, Thames and Hudson.

Morris, M. (1990), Mystery identity of 1959 HIV case, *The Guardian*, 7 July, Home page, 4.

Mulvey, L. (1973), Fears, fantasies and the male unconscious or 'You don't know what is happening, do you, Mr Jones?', in *Visual and Other Pleasures*, London, Macmillan, 1989.

Namjoshi, S. (1991), I give her the rose, in J. Barrington (ed.), *An Intimate Wilderness: Lesbian Writers on Sexuality*, Portland, Eighth Mountain Press.

Nast, H. J. and A. Kobayashi (1996), Re-corporealizing vision, in N. Duncan (ed.), *Body Space*, London, Routledge.

Neil, A. (1993), Letter: Aids and the Sunday Times, *The Guardian*, 17 December, Features, 23.

Newtown, G. (1989), Sex, death, and the drama of AIDS, *The Antioch Review*, 47/2, 209–22.

Nightingale, B. (1993), More in sorrow than in anger, *The Times*, 24 September.

Ochert, A. (1999), Cresting controversy, *Times Higher Educational Supplement*, 23 April 1999. Features section. Version 31 July. <http://www.thesis.co.uk>

Odets, W. (1997), Why we do not do primary prevention for gay men, in J. Oppenheimer and H. Reckitt (eds), *Acting on AIDS: Sex, Drugs and Politics*, London, Serpent's Tail.

Oppenheimer, J. (1997), Movements, markets, and the mainstream: gay activism and assimilation in the age of AIDS, in O'Flaherty, M. (1983), Expert refuses 'AIDS death' probe, *Daily Express* 2 November.

Oppenheimer, J. and H. Reckitt (eds) (1997), *Acting on AIDS: Sex, Drugs and Politics*, London, Serpent's Tail.

O'Pray, M. (1996), The art of films/films of art, in R. Wollen (ed.), *Derek Jarman: A Portrait*, London, Thames and Hudson.

O'Sullivan, S. (1990), Mapping: lesbianism, AIDS, and sexuality, *Feminist Review*, 34, 120–33.

Park, K. (1993), Kimberly Bergalis, AIDS, and the plague metaphor, in M. Garber, J. Matlock and R. L. Walkowitz (eds), *Media Spectacles*, London, Routledge, 1993.

Parker, A., Russo, M., Sommer, D. and P. Yaeger (eds) (1992), *Nationalisms and Sexualities*, London, Routledge.

Parkes, J. C. (1996), Sexuality and the gay sensibility, in R. Wollen (ed.), *Derek Jarman: A Portrait*, London, Thames and Hudson.

Pass notes No. 295 (1993): Aids, *The Guardian*, 30 November, G2T, 3.

Patton, C. (1997), Queer peregrinations, in J. Oppenheimer and H. Reckitt (eds), *Acting on AIDS: Sex, Drugs and Politics*, London, Serpent's Tail.

Patton, C. (1996), *Fatal Advice: How Safe-sex Education Went Wrong*, Durham, Duke University Press.

Patton, C. (1995), Performativity and spatial distinction, in A. Parker and E. Kosofsky Sedgwick (eds), *Performativity and Performance*, London, Routledge.

Patton, C. (1990), *Inventing AIDS*, London, Routledge.

Patton, C. (1989), The AIDS industry: construction of 'victims', 'volunteers' and 'experts', in E. Carter and S. Watney (eds), *Taking Liberties: AIDS and Cultural Politics*, London, Serpent's Tail.

Pazè, E. (1998), 12th world AIDS conference, *The Lancet*, 352, 26 September, 1072.

Phelan, P. (1997), *Mourning Sex: Performing Public Memories*, London, Routledge.

Phelan, P. (1993), *Unmarked: The Politics of Performance*, London, Routledge.

Philadelphia (1993), dir. J. Demme, Tristar Pictures.

Phoolcharoen, W. (1999), HIV vaccines for southeast Asia and south Asia: the challenges and opportunities, Version 27 July 1999. <http://www.hsph.harvard.edu/hai/conferences/thailand_reports/thailand-1996-3.html>

Picture of the week (1997), *The Guardian*, 27 September, 2.

Piontek, T. (1992), Unsafe representations: cultural criticism in the age of AIDS, *Discourse*, 15/1, 128–53.

Piscator, E. (1929, rpt 1979), *Das Politische Theater*, Hamburg, Rowohlt Verlag.

Plasai, V. (1993), Letter: The awful consequences of unlimited sex, *The Guardian*, 3 December, Features, 25.

Pollock, G. (1988), *Vision and Difference: Femininity, Feminism and the Histories of Art*, London, Routledge.

Positive Women Victoria Inc. (1999), Women like us. Version 27 July 1999. <http://www.home.aone.net.au/pos.women/text/us.html>

Powell, R. (1995), Fifty-plus and face to face with AIDS, *The Independent*, 9 January, LIFE, 19.

Price, J. and M. Shildrick (eds) (1999), *Feminist Theory and the Body*, Edinburgh, Edinburgh University Press.

Radford, J. (ed.) (1986), *The Progress of Romance*, London, Routledge and Kegan Paul.

Radford, J. and D. E. H. Russell (eds) (1992), *Femicide: The Politics of Woman Killing*, Buckingham, Open University Press.

Radford, T. (1996), Influence and power of the media, *The Lancet*, 347, 1 June, 1533-5.

Radicalesbians (1970), The woman identified woman, in S. L. Hoagland and J. Penelope (eds), *For Lesbians Only*, London, Onlywomen Press, 1988.

Radway, J. (1987), *Reading the Romance*, London, Verso.

Rich, A. (1980), Compulsory heterosexuality and lesbian existence, in A. Snitow, C. Stansell and S. Thompson (eds), *Desire: The Politics of Sexuality*, London, Virago, 1983.

Richardson, D. (1994a), AIDS: Issues for feminism in the UK, in L. Doyal, J. Naidoo and T. Wilton (eds), *AIDS: Setting a Feminist Agenda*, London, Taylor & Francis.

Richardson, D. (1994b), Inclusions and exclusions: lesbians, HIV and AIDS, in L. Doyal, J. Naidoo and T. Wilton (eds), *AIDS: Setting a Feminist Agenda*, London, Taylor & Francis.

Richardson, D. (1987), *Women and the AIDS Crisis*, London, Pandora.

Rieder, I. and P. Ruppelt (eds) (1989), *Matters of Life and Death: Women Speak About AIDS*, London, Virago.

Roth, N. L. and L. K. Fuller (eds) (1998), *Women and AIDS: Negotiating Safer Practices, Care, and Prevention*, New York, Harrington Park Press.

Roth, N. L. and K. Hogan (eds) (1998), *Gendered Epidemic: Representations of Women in the Age of AIDS*, London, Routledge.

Roxan, D. (1984), Nurses in AIDS threat told to work on, *News of the World*, 8 January.

Rubin, G. (1988), Thinking sex: notes of a radical theory of the politics of sexuality, in C.S. Vance (ed.), *Pleasure and Danger: Exploring Female Sexuality*, London, Pandora.

Rushing, W. (1995), *The AIDS Epidemic*, Boulder, Colorado, Westview Press.

Ruskin, C. (1988), *The Quilt: Stories from the NAMES Project*, New York, Pocket Books.

Russian, D. A. and J. A. Kovacs (1995), Pneumocystis carinii in Africa: an emerging pathogen?, *The Lancet*, 346, 11 November, 1242.

Saalfield, C. and R. Navarro (1991), Shocking pink praxis: race and gender on the ACT UP frontlines, in D. Fuss (ed.), *Inside/Out: Lesbian Theories, Gay Theories*, London, Routledge.

Sabatier, R. (1988), *Blaming Others: Prejudice, Race and Worldwide AIDS*, London, Panos Institute.

Said, E. W. (1993), *Culture and Imperialism*, London, Chatto and Windus.

Said, E. W. (1978), *Orientalism*, London, Penguin.

Sarsby, J. (1983), *Romantic Love and Society*, Harmondsworth, Penguin.

Schwartz, R. (1993), New alliances, strange bedfellows: lesbians, gay men, and AIDS, in A. Stein (ed.), *Sisters, Sexperts, Queers*, New York, Plume.

Schwenger, P. (1996), Derek Jarman and the colour of the mind's eye, *University of Toronto Quarterly*, 65/2, 419–26.

Scott, P. (1997), White noise: how gay men's activism gets written out of AIDS prevention, in J. Oppenheimer and H. Reckitt (eds), *Acting on AIDS: Sex, Drugs and Politics*, London, Serpent's Tail.

Sedgwick, E. K. (1985), *Between Men: English Literature and Male Homosocial Desire*, New York, Columbia University Press.

Sedgwick, E. K. (1990; rpt 1994), *Epistemology of the Closet*, London, Penguin.

Selden, D. L. (1995), 'Just when you thought it was safe to go back in the water …', in N. Blake, L. Rinder and A. Scholder (eds), *In a Different Light: Visual Culture, Sexual Identity, Queer Practice*, San Francisco, City Lights Books.

Sheba Collective (eds) (1989), *Serious Pleasure*, London, Sheba Feminist Publishers.

Sheiner, M. (1999), *Herotica 6*, San Francisco, Down There Press.

Sherman, J. (1990), Fostering guidelines, *The Times on CDRom*, 30 January, n. p.

Shildrick, M. (1997), *Leaky Bodies and Boundaries*, London, Routledge.

Shilts, R. (1987), *And the Band Played On: Politics, People, and the AIDS Epidemic*, rpt London, Penguin, 1988.

Showalter, E. (1991), *Sexual Anarchy: Gender and Culture at the Fin de Siècle*, London, Bloomsbury.

Silverman, K. (1996), *The Threshold of the Visible World*, London, Routledge.

Singer, L. (1993), *Erotic Welfare: Sexual Theory and Politics in the Age of Epidemic*, London, Routledge.

Smith, A. M. (1994), *New Right Discourse on Race and Sexuality*, Cambridge, Cambridge University Press.

Sontag, S. (1988), *AIDS and Its Metaphors*, New York, Farrar, Straus and Giroux.

Spence, J. (1995), *Cultural Sniping: The Art of Transgression*, London, Routledge.

Spence, J. (1987), *Putting Myself in the Picture*, London, Camden.

Squiers, C. (ed.) (1990), *The Critical Image: Essays on Contemporary Photography*, Seattle, Bay Press.

Stacey, J. (1997), *Teratologies: A Cultural Study of Cancer*, London, Routledge.

Stein, A. (ed.) (1993), *Sisters, Sexperts, Queers*, New York, Plume.

Steinem, G. (1980), Erotica and pornography: a clear and present difference, in L. Lederer (ed.), *Take Back the Night: Women and Pornography*, New York, William Morrow and Co.

Stewart, G. (1999), The great Aids pandemic, *Times Higher Educational Supplement*, 21 May 1999. Features section. Version 31 July 1999. <http://www.thesis.co.uk>

Stone, A. R. (1996), *The War Between Desire and Technology at the Close of the Mechanical Age*, Cambridge, MA, MIT Press.

Sturrock, J. (1993), The estate – a family secret, in S. Mayes and L. Stein (eds), *Positive Lives*, London, Cassell.

Svede, M. A. (1989), What's happened here, in J. Z. Grover (ed.), *AIDS: The Artists' Response*, Columbus, Hoyt L. Sherman Gallery.

Taormino, T. (1999), *Best Lesbian Erotica 1999*, San Francisco, Cleis Press.

Taylor, H. (1989), Romantic readers, in H. Carr, *From My Guy to Sci Fi*, London, Pandora.

Taylor, P. (1996), Ten Years in the arts: *Angels in America*: the play that gave the stage a new direction, *Independent* 11 October, Features, 8, 9.

Thornber, R. (1993), The destiny of me, *The Guardian*, 23 September.

Tisdall, S. (1993), Horror's homeland, *The Guardian*, 30 October, Weekend, 4.

Torres, L. (1993), AIDS refusniks, *The Guardian*, 11 December, 35.

Treichler, P. (1997), How to use a condom: lessons from the AIDS epidemic, in J. Oppenheimer and H. Reckitt (eds), *Acting on AIDS: Sex, Drugs and Politics*, London, Serpent's Tail.

Treichler, P. (1993), AIDS narratives on television: whose story?, in T. F. Murphy and S. Poirier (eds), *Writing AIDS*, New York, Columbia University Press, 1993.

Treichler, P. (1991), AIDS, homophobia, and biomedical discourse: an epidemic of signification, in D. Crimp (ed.), *AIDS: Cultural Analysis, Cultural Activism*, Cambridge, MA, MIT Press, 1991.

Treichler, P. (1989), AIDS and HIV infection in the third world: a first world chronicle, in B. Kruger and P. Mariani (eds), *Remaking History*, Seattle, Bay Press.

Treichler, P. (1988), AIDS, gender, and biomedical discourse, in E. Fee, and D. M. Fox (eds), *AIDS: The Burdens of History*, Berkeley, University of California Press.

Tsui, K. (1992), Who says we don't talk about sex?, in J. Nestle (ed.), *The Persistent Desire: A Butch–Femme Reader*, Boston, Alyson Press.

Turner, B. (1994), Preface, in P. Falk, *The Consuming Body*, London, Sage.

Tyler, C.-A. (1997), Passing: narcissism, identity, and difference, in E. Weed and N. Schor (eds), *Feminism Meets Queer Theory*, Bloomington, Indiana University Press, 227–65.

Ughetto, B. (1993), *Images pour la Lutte Contre le SIDA – Images Against AIDS*, Paris, Artis.

UK NGO AIDS Consortium (1998), Access to treatment for HIV in developing countries, *The Lancet*, 352, 24 October, 1379–80.

UNAIDS/WHO (1998), *Global HIV/AIDS and STD Surveillance: AIDS Epidemic Update, December 1998*. Version 10 June 1999. <http:www.unaids.org/unaids/document/epidemio/dec98/global%5Freport/index.html>

Valdiserri, R. O. (1994) *Gardening in Clay: Reflections on AIDS*, Ithaca, Cornell University Press.

Valverde, M. (1985), *Sex, Power and Pleasure*, London, Women's Press.

Vance, C. (1994), The war on culture, in T. Gott (ed.), *Don't Leave Me This Way: Art in the Age of AIDS*, Melbourne, Thames and Hudson, 1994.

Vazquez, C. (1998), The good and the bad, in N. L. Roth and K. Hogan (eds), *Gendered Epidemic: Representations of Women in the Age of AIDS*, London, Routledge.

Waldby, C. (1996), *AIDS and the Body Politic: Biomedicine and Sexual Difference*, London, Routledge.

Walker, M. (1990), Kinsey finds US sexually illiterate, *Guardian*, 6 September 1990: 20.

Wallerstein, C. (1998), Philippines finally passes AIDS act, *The Lancet*, 351, 7 March, 734.

Watney, S. (1999), HIV–AIDS link irrefutable, *Times Higher Educational Supplement*, 21 May. Letters section. Version 31 July 1999. <http://www.thesis.co.uk>

Watney, S. (1997), The political significance of statistics in the AIDS crisis: epidemiology, representation and re-gaying, in J. Oppenheimer and H. Reckitt (eds), *Acting on AIDS: Sex, Drugs and Politics*, London, Serpent's Tail.

Watney, S. (1994), *Practices of Freedom: Selected Writings on HIV/AIDS*, London, Rivers Oram Press.

Watney, S. (1992), Seeing AIDS: the work of Brian Weil, in B. Weil, *Every 17 Seconds*, New York, Aperture Foundation Inc.

Watney, S. (1991), The spectacle of AIDS, in D. Crimp (ed.), *AIDS: Cultural Analysis Cultural Activism*, Cambridge, MA, MIT Press.

Watney, S. (1990a), Representing AIDS, in T. Boffin and S. Gupta (eds), *Ecstatic Antibodies: Resisting the AIDS Mythology*, London, Rivers Oram Press, 1990.

Watney, S. (1990b), Photography and AIDS, in C. Squiers (ed.), *The Critical Image: Essays on Contemporary Photography*, Seattle, Bay Press.

Watney, S. (1989/90), Bodies of experience, *Ten 8*, /35 (winter) 17–18.

Watney, S. (1989a), Taking liberties: an introduction, in E. Carter and S. Watney (eds) (1989), *Taking Liberties: AIDS and Cultural Politics*, London, Serpent's Tail.

Watney, S. (1989b), AIDS, language and the third world, in E. Carter and S. Watney (eds), *Taking Liberties: AIDS and Cultural Politics*, London, Serpent's Tail.

Watney, S. (1987), *Policing Desire: Pornography, AIDS and the Media*, London, Methuen.

Watson, S. (1995), Erotophobia: a forum on sexuality, in N. Blake, L. Rinder and A. Scholder (eds), *In a Different Light: Visual Culture, Sexual Identity, Queer Practice*, San Francisco, City Lights Books.

Weed, E. and N. Schor (eds) (1997), *Feminism Meets Queer Theory*, Bloomington, Indiana University Press.

Weeks, J. (1990), Post-modern AIDS?, in T. Boffin and S. Gupta (eds), *Ecstatic Antibodies: Resisting the AIDS Mythology*, London, Rivers Oram Press.

Wellings, K. and B. Field (1996), *Stopping AIDS*, Harlow, Longman.

Wellings, K. Field, J., Johnson, A. M. and J. Wadsworth (1994), *Sexual Behaviour in Britain: The National Survey of Sexual Attitudes and Lifestyles*, Harmondsworth, Penguin.

Whatever Happened to the Plague? (1999), Channel 4, 3 January, 7.55pm–9.30pm.

Whisman, V. (1993), Identity crisis: who is a lesbian anyway?, in A. Stein (ed.), *Sisters, Sexperts, Queers*, New York, Plume.

White, E. (1994), Aesthetics and loss, in T. Gott (ed.), *Don't Leave Me This Way: Art in the Age of AIDS*, Melbourne, Thames & Hudson, 1994.

White, H. (1978), *Tropics of Discourse*, Baltimore, Johns Hopkins University Press.

White, H. (1973), *Metahistory*, Baltimore, Johns Hopkins University Press.

Whitehead, T. (1989), The voluntary sector: five years on, in E. Carter and S. Watney (eds), *Taking Liberties: AIDS and Cultural Politics*, London, Serpent's Tail, 1989.

Williamson, J. (1989), Every virus tells a story: the meanings of HIV and AIDS, in E. Carter and S. Watney (eds) (1989), *Taking Liberties: AIDS and Cultural Politics*, London, Serpent's Tail.

Wilton, T. (1997), *Engendering AIDS: Deconstructing Sex, Text and Epidemic*, London, Sage.

Wilton, T. (1994), Feminism and the erotics of health promotion, in L. Doyal, J. Naidoo and T. Wilton (eds), *AIDS: Setting a Feminist Agenda*, London, Taylor & Francis.

Wilton, T. (1992), *Antibody Politic: AIDS and Society*, Cheltenham, New Clarion Press.

Wittig, M. (1992), One is not born a woman, in *The Straight Mind and Other Essays*, London, Harvester Wheatsheaf.

Wojnarowicz, D. (1991), *Close to the Knives: A Memoir of Disintegration*, New York, Vintage Books.

Wolffers, I. and I. Fernandez (1995), Migration and AIDS, *The Lancet*, 346, 11 November, 1303.

Wollen, R. (ed.) (1996), *Derek Jarman: A Portrait*, London, Thames and Hudson.

Woods, G. (1992), AIDS to remembrance: the uses of elegy, in E. S. Nelson (ed.), *AIDS: The Literary Response*, New York, Twayne Publishers.

Wu, Z., Liu, Z. and R. Detels (1995), HIV-1 infection in commercial plasma donors in China, *The Lancet*, 346, 1 July, 61–2.

Yingling, T. (1994), Wittgenstein's tumor: AIDS and the national body, *Textual Practice*, 8, 97–113.

Yingling, T. (1991), Acting up: AIDS, allegory, activism, in D. Fuss (ed.), *Inside/Out: Lesbian Theories, Gay Theories*, London, Routledge, 1991.

Young, R. (ed.) (1981), *Untying the Text* London, Routledge.

Zhu, T. and D. Ho (1995), Was HIV present in 1959? *Nature*, 374, 503–5.

Zivi, K. (1998), Constituting the 'clean and proper' body: convergences between abjection and AIDS, in N. L. Roth and K. Hogan (eds), *Gendered Epidemic: Representations of Women in the Age of AIDS*, London, Routledge.

Index

Note: 'n.' after a page reference indicates a note number on that page.